What the world needs now is *Christian Psychiatry*

Mental health problems are afflicting more Americans today than ever before; suicide is a leading cause of death in the United States. Despite the upsurge of interest in the field of counseling and the vast increase in expenditures and research designed to solve the problem, the situation continues to worsen. There must be another way.

Drs. Frank Minirth and Walter Byrd offer an alternative to the limited "secular solution" — *Christian Psychiatry*. They define Christian counseling as "the ministry of one individual seeking to help another individual recognize, understand, and solve his own problems in accordance with the Word of God." This informative and enlightening book explores the spiritual dimension, combining proven scientific truth with the foundational truths of the Bible, recognizing "the dependence on not only man's willpower to be responsible, but also on God's enabling, indwelling power of the Holy Spirit to conquer man's problems."

CHRISTIAN PSYCHIATRY

FRANK B. MINIRTH, M.D. AND WALTER BYRD, M.D.

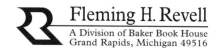
Fleming H. Revell
A Division of Baker Book House
Grand Rapids, Michigan 49516

All case studies used in this book are composites.

Library of Congress Cataloging in Publication Data

Minirth, Frank B.
  Christian psychiatry.

  Bibliography: p.
  Includes index.
  1. Psychiatry and religion. I. Title.
RC455.4.R4M56 1977   616.8′9   76-57767
ISBN 0-8007-5352-6

TO Mary Alice, who is my wife, companion, and friend. Her love and encouragement have made this book possible.

Frank Minirth, M.D.

TO my wife, Karen, who is my love, my friend, and my tireless encourager.

Walt Byrd, M.D.

Contents

Introduction

Christian Psychiatry, does it exist? Is there such a field of thinking? Can Christianity and psychiatry coexist? We believe there is such a philosophy and in this book have developed the concepts we've chosen to simply describe as Christian Psychiatry. Not only can the concept apply to Christians within the psychiatric profession, but to Christian counselors in general. In fact, the principles should help not only counselors but laymen as well.

In Christian Psychiatry the counselor is concerned not only with psychological and physical problems, but also with spiritual problems, whereas in other approaches to counseling, sometimes the spiritual aspect of man is, unfortunately, not addressed. In Christian Psychiatry the counselor is concerned with understanding the psychological makeup of man and how psychodynamic factors have impacted on each individual's functioning. In Christian Psychiatry the counselor is aware that physical problems may be contributing to an apparent spiritual or psychological problem. In other words, a balanced Christian counseling approach should deal with the whole man.

In Christian Psychiatry the whole foundation revolves around the nature of man and especially how man's nature is revealed through the truths contained in Scripture. The Bible gives a Christian counselor a foundation, stability, and guidelines as he

11

or she approaches the problems that face the individual. In Christian Psychiatry the supernatural is felt to make a definite difference, whereas in some secular schools it is generally ignored. Prayer, Bible study, and the power of the Holy Spirit within an individual are seen as resources that can be applied frequently to effectively assist the individual in obtaining a more productive and healthy life.

In Christian Psychiatry the counselor seeks a balance without focusing either entirely on the past or only on the present, and without focusing either entirely on feelings or only on behavior. Christian Psychiatry strives to be practical, focusing on useful ways of recognizing spiritual problems and practical ways of recognizing psychological problems, as well as understanding the role physical problems can play in affecting a person's mental function as well.

In Christian Psychiatry valid psychiatric knowledge is felt to be important. Although the Christian counselor certainly holds the Scriptures to be valid and wholly truthful, he does not treat proven scientific truth as invalid. Thus, Christian Psychiatry is unique for several reasons and it exists as a valuable philosophy for helping individuals suffering from emotional and mental disorders. In the past decade, the field of Christian Psychiatry has greatly increased, with many Christians receiving help medically, psychologically, and spiritually.

Frank Minirth, M.D.
Walter Byrd, M.D.
March 1990

For further information regarding
the nationwide services of the
Minirth-Meier Clinic, please call

1/800/NEW LIFE (Clinical Services)
or
1/800/BOOKS-4-LIFE
(National Resources Division)

Part I

An Introduction to Christian Psychiatry

> The Lord God hath given me the
> tongue of the learned, that I should
> know how to speak a word in season
> to him that is weary. . . .
>
> ISAIAH 50:4

> The above words are so applicable to
> Christian counselors today. They
> were written centuries ago by the
> Prophet Isaiah and pertain to the
> Counselor of counselors—Jesus
> Christ.
>
> THE AUTHORS

1 Why Christian Psychiatry?

Recently a gentleman named Robert made an appointment to see one of the doctors at our clinic. He complained that everyone had forsaken him. While talking with him, it became apparent that Robert had a gradually worsening mental problem that was making it hard for him to relate to other people. One could easily see why his wife, his children, and even his friends eventually gave up the struggle of trying to relate to him. He also reported that, despite everyone's forsaking him, a few years ago he had found Someone who never forsakes him, Jesus Christ.

This man typifies the need for the practice of Christian psychiatry, treating the whole person—physically, psychologically, and spiritually. After a thorough evaluation it was evident that Robert had a need not only for medical help to overcome a chemical imbalance in his brain, but also for mental and behavioral help in learning how to realistically view and behave around other people. The stress of each problem had made the other worse, not an unusual situation. The fact that Robert knew Jesus Christ as his personal Savior would prove to be an important part of his treatment.

Man's frustration in dealing with life's problems is no new phenomenon. In fact, counseling has been important to mankind since the beginning of time. Many have looked to seers and to the stars for advice. "Wise men" were consulted by kings to

15

interpret dreams and to give them advice on matters pertaining to business, love, and death. In relatively recent times, counseling has become a full-fledged profession, with many states now requiring licensure

Emotional Problems—Inside and Outside the Church

Because of the increased knowledge of the importance of mental health in recent years, and because of our willingness to talk about mental problems rather than hide them away in the attic, there has been an upsurge of interest in the field of counseling. Man wants to know why he and others behave as they do. The depressed person is uncomfortable and wants to know what he can do for relief. Another person suffers from the anguish of guilt. What can he do to rid himself of this burden? Parents want to know the best way to raise their children and wonder why their adolescent is so rebellious. The adolescent believes he sees through the "facade" of adults and is skeptical, but he, too, is confused and wants to understand himself. It is not surprising that many, many books in the field of counseling and child development have become best-sellers.

We Christians are not immune to the pressures of today's hectic pace, and more and more the Christian community is becoming interested in counseling. To this end, in the past decade many skillful Christian counselors have written books in an attempt to help Christian men and women understand their behavior and solve their particular problems.

Many Christians want to know *if*, in fact, they should even have problems. An individual recently asked if a Christian could become a schizophrenic. What's more, Christians want to know *why* they should seek help. Some muse over the relationship between doubts concerning their salvation, anxiety, and their personality types. Some Christians wonder why their illicit sexual urges are so strong. They feel frustrated and ashamed, and they ask what they can do. They want to understand why they find themselves so easily entangled in unhealthy "co-dependent" relationships. These and other questions and problems are shared by very many Christians.

This world of ours is moving at a tremendously rapid pace, and we as Christians, sensitive to those in the world, will continue to find that we are not immune to this insidious affliction.

The Secular Solution

The stress and emotional pressure upon individuals is staggering, and to help meet the demands of psychological problems, new and practical psychotherapeutic techniques have been developed over the years. Although they do not claim to be Christian, some of the approaches contain principles found within the Scriptures. For example, the approach called *Reality Therapy* is based on being responsible, facing reality, and doing what is right. *Cognitive Therapy* stresses that transforming change comes through renewing the mind and its thought patterns.

In brief, secular psychotherapy could be broken down into seven schools of thought.[1]

The first of these is the school centering around the *Psychoanalytic Theory*. Sigmund Freud developed this theory in the early 1900s. It is based on the stages of development of man (oral, anal, oedipal, and latent), a structure of personality (*id*, *ego*, and *superego*), and a technique of solving unresolved, unconscious conflicts. This theory focuses on the impact of the dynamic unconscious on behavior. The emphasis is on individual introspection and the technique is "free association," whereby one discusses whatever comes to his mind. The therapist, in turn, listens, makes comments at times, and hopes to help the patient work through conflicts that originated in his infantile years. Therapy may require hundreds of hours. This school has received much criticism, especially from the religious community, because it has not emphasized personal responsibility. Also, because it does not deal with the spiritual aspect of man, it offers no effective way to deal with true guilt. Many ministers believe that most psychiatrists are of this school; however, only 10 percent of the psychiatrists in this country are psychoanalysts.[2]

The next theory to influence the new science of psychology is known as the *Neo-psychoanalytic* (or *Interpersonal*) *Theory* of psychology. According to this theory, man is a product of society, and his personality is determined more by social factors than by biologic ones.[3] The founders of this school had originally been friends and colleagues of Freud but split with him over the importance of social factors. They felt that Freud had largely neglected the social influence on man's development. These theorists include Alfred Adler, Karen Horney, Erich Fromm, and Harry Stack Sullivan.

Alfred Adler was the first to emphasize the importance of social factors in personality development. Where Freud emphasized biological factors, inborn instincts, and sexual drive, Adler emphasized social influences.[4] Where Freud emphasized the impact of sexual drives on behavior, Adler again emphasized social influences.[5] Both assumed man had inherent factors that affected his destiny, but for Adler, those factors were social.[6]

The third school of thought centers around a practical, commonsense approach called *Reality Therapy*, developed by William Glasser. This theory is based on the value of "doing right," facing reality, and being responsible. These therapists focus on the present, not the past, and on behavior, not feelings. They help man to work out practical solutions to his problems. This theory states that people in need of psychiatric treatment suffer from failing to fulfill two basic needs in life—love and self-worth. In contrast to conventional therapy, they do not look for unconscious conflicts, nor do they permit the patient to excuse his behavior on the basis of unconscious conflicts. Furthermore, they do affirm the morality of behavior. They, in contrast to conventional therapy, attempt to distinguish between right and wrong. This is commendable, but, because of their secular perspective, their definition of morality is relative. This school of thought has affected Christian counselors prominently. For example, Jay Adams, one of the best known of Christian counselors, spent significant time in training with Orval Hobart Mowrer, a founder of Reality Therapy. This is evident in his writings. Also, Paul Morris, who wrote *Love Therapy*, included a chapter on Reality Therapy. In a related genre, Carl Rogers, a former seminary student, developed a very widely used approach called the "self-directed approach." He emphasized individuals accepting responsibility for meeting their own needs based on the value and worth of the individual, disregarding the concept of the depravity of man.

The fourth school of thought was originated by Eric Berne in the 1950s and 1960s. This school is known as *Transactional Analysis* or TA. This school of thought is based on three ego states in man: parent, adult, and child. These therapists state that in our transactions with others, we always relate on one of these three levels. This is a responsibility-oriented and goal-oriented therapy, and much emphasis is also placed on the importance of giving "strokes" or encouragement and recognition to others. Some therapists have combined the TA concepts with another school of thought called the Gestalt School. This combination appears to have practical application in some cases.

The founder of TA, Eric Berne, became best known to the public for his book *Games People Play*. In this book, Berne wrote of such games as "Mine is better than yours," "Ain't it awful," "If it were not for you," "Kick me," "I'm only trying to help you," and "Why don't you yes but." The "games" are essentially patterns of deed and thought, by which an individual tries to manipulate others. Unfortunately, Christians can become equally skillful at such unhealthy games.

Other TA authors have emphasized what they would call "life-basic" positions. Many people have read *I'm OK—You're OK*. In this book, Thomas Harris denoted the criminal position as "I'm OK—You're not OK," the position of the depressive as "I'm not OK—You're OK," and the healthy position as "I'm OK—You're OK." These thoughts are not without merit and may sometimes be useful in understanding why certain persons continually see relationships through long-standing distorted perceptions.

The fifth school of thought is known as *Behavior Modification*. These therapists stress overt behavior and conditioning responses. This school had its beginning with a Russian physiologist, Ivan Pavlov, who demonstrated a conditioned response in his famous experiments with a dog. Such men as Joseph Wolpe, J. B. Watson, and B. F. Skinner have pursued this school of thought, where emphasis is on positive reinforcement, negative reinforcement, desensitization, reciprocal inhibition, conditioned avoidance, and the concept of extinction. Examples of its use today include smoking cessation, weight control, and management of phobias.

The sixth school of thought is referred to as *Cognitive Therapy*. This approach was largely formulated by Aaron Beck of the University of Pennsylvania. This therapy operates upon the premise that within our minds a sequence occurs as follows: Initial perceptions are received, these perceptions become cognitive thoughts, and then emotions subsequently arise from these cognitive thoughts. The Cognitive Therapy for depression holds that, if a person can change the self-defeating and negative thought processes (cognitions) to healthier ones, then the negative emotions will change as well. David Burns, M.D., in his book, *Feeling Good, The New Mood Therapy*, championed this form of therapy. It has been found useful for treating depression. Dr. Albert Ellis has for years espoused a similar form of treatment that he calls Rational Emotive Therapy. The ABC theory states that events give rise to thoughts (beliefs) that lead to emotions, and a person can control his emotions by eliminating unhealthy and irrational beliefs and thoughts.

The seventh school of thought concerning treatment has just recently come into its own, although it has been around for years. It is the *Twelve-Step Movement*. The Twelve-Step approach was originally developed within Alcoholics Anonymous to help those afflicted recover from alcoholism. However, the application of the Twelve-Step format has been utilized with a wide variety of disorders, including co-dependency, adult children of alcoholics, overeating, gambling addiction, sexual addiction, incest recovery, and narcotics addiction. On any given evening, tens of thousands of people are involved in twelve-step groups of one type or another throughout the United States. Twelve-Step groups acknowledge the need for a higher power than man himself to be called upon for true recovery to occur, but only Christian Twelve-Step groups specifically identify that higher power as Jesus Christ.

Why a Non-Christian Approach Is Limited

The therapists from these secular schools of human behavior have given us much scientific information. We have learned, for instance, that we all have certain defenses by which we handle stress. Some of these defense mechanisms are healthy and some are unhealthy. *Sublimation* can be a healthy subconscious defense mechanism when one handles anxiety by sublimating it in some productive direction, but *denial* can be an unhealthy subconscious defense mechanism whereby one fails to recognize obvious facts or implications.

We have learned, further, that social factors are definitely important in a person's psychological makeup. There is little doubt that much of the basic personality trend is set by age six. Such individual characteristics as being perfectionistic, dramatic, withdrawn, explosive, and passive are developed early and are largely determined by the social and familial factors around us. Of course, this is not to say that the Lord cannot change people, but rather that their personality strengths and weaknesses are determined at an early age. Once a person accepts Christ, the Lord works both through other Christians and through His Word to strengthen the positive trends in one's personality and overcome the weaknesses.

We have also learned that psychiatry can be practical. We can help people face reality and be responsible. We can help them find practical solutions to their problems. We can help them through our scientific observation and their own insight to understand how they are relating to others and how they may need to change in order to be more adult and mature. Through clinical studies, we have learned about the importance of such techniques as behavior modification and how the proper treatment of chemical imbalances in the brain can be remarkably effective.

Yet, while some of these approaches are very practical and may be quite helpful, they have limitations. First, there is no standard of authority besides man's logic or conscience. To be sure, man's logic is a poor standard of authority because a man can subconsciously use logic to justify what he wishes. Neither is man's conscience a good standard, for his conscience develops mostly during his first five years of life from exposure to his parents and their morals. Therefore, a man brought up by overly strict parents would possess a rigid conscience. Conversely, a man brought up by sociopathic parents would suffer from an undeveloped conscience. In Proverbs 16:25, King Solomon recorded, "There is a way that seemeth right unto a man, but the end thereof are the ways of death." In Judges 21:25, the author wrote, "In those days there was no king in Israel: every man did that which was right in his own eyes." It is an understatement to say that the end of this course of following man's conscience alone was less than healthy for the nation of Israel.

Second, the application of some of the new approaches depends on man's own willpower. On the one hand, the founders of these new approaches are to be commended for forcing psychiatry to recognize that man has a free will and is responsible for his actions, but, on the other hand, this idea can be carried to an extreme, whereby man alone has the capability within himself to solve all his problems. We as Christians know that man's willpower can prove insufficient according to Apostle Paul in Romans 7. (*See* Romans 7:18.)

Third, most of these approaches do not address the fact that man, when left to his own ends, tends to be basically selfish and sinful. Thus, any approach could be subject to conscious and subconscious attempts by the individual to utilize the method to perpetuate a narrow, self-centered view of life, thereby ultimately avoiding the deeper need of the individual to become spiritually whole and enter a right relationship with God through Jesus Christ.

The Christian Solution

Christian counselors are also trying to help meet the demands of emotional problems. Inasmuch as so many turn to ministers for counsel (42 percent of the people who seek counsel turn to their ministers),[7] a review of the field of Christian counseling in general would be helpful at this point.

Many professionals have written about religion and psychiatry in general.[8-25] Some have also written specifically about Christianity and psychiatry. Freud was not impressed with the beliefs of religion in general or Christianity in particular. In fact, he felt it was a "universal, obsessional neurosis."[26] Jung, on the other hand, felt religion was very important, and he wrote much in the field of religion and psychiatry.[27] Of course, the work of William James, *The Varieties of Religious Experience*, has become a classic.[28] As Adler's and Fromm's major contributions have been in this field, they apparently felt it played an important part in man's life and psychological makeup.[29, 30] Lesser known theorists such as Christensen and Allison felt that religious conversion might help to reintegrate a weakened ego, and Pattison felt that there might be validity for the claim that the therapist should help the patient work toward spiritual goals.[31–33] In the same manner, Bronner and Bergman believed there should be a positive acceptance or respect for the patient's religious beliefs.[34, 35] Meyerson has presented a provocative psychoanalytic meaning of the Cross. He feels that it is not only a symbol of Christianity and the crucifixion, but also of love, since a person with arms outstretched represents tenderness, warmth, affection, and a readiness to embrace.[36] He has further suggested that a person terrified by love would try to destroy this symbol. And finally, classic papers by Wilson and Nicoli (Christian psychiatrists) have pointed out the positive benefits of religious conversion, citing improved impulse control, improved academic performance, and improved interpersonal relationships as evidence that religious conversion may be one of the most profoundly transforming of human experiences.[37–39]

However, the major contributions to Christian counseling generally have not come from the professionals listed above (many of whom were not Christians), but from Christian counselors themselves. Gary Collins, psychologist and professor at Liberty University, has divided Christian counselors into five main categories, including the "mainstream," the evangelical pastoral counselors, the Christian professional, the theoretician-researcher, and the "popularizers."[40]

Categories of Christian Counselors

Mainstream counselors are a large source of current training in pastoral psychology and counseling.[41] This source is the Clinical Pastoral Education (CPE) movement, a movement which is highly organized and which has done much commendable work with counseling curricula in hospitals and seminaries. However, this movement has drawn some criticism from conservative evangelicals for possibly being too liberal, and some in the movement put human experience and psychology above the Word of God.[42] Anton Boiser was one of the founders of the CPE movement. Other familiar names involved in CPE are Seward Hiltner, Edward Thornton, and Russell Dicks.

The second category is the *Evangelical Pastoral* counselors, a group which is made up, obviously, of evangelical pastors and ministers. They are firmly committed to a sound biblical source for all counseling, and many of them counsel through excellent preaching/teaching on personal problems from the pulpit. These would include men such as Charles Swindol, Charles Stanley, D. James Kennedy, and John MacArthur. Jay Adams was one of the forerunners in this group, and, although he is perceived by some as being more antagonistic toward the M.D. and Ph.D. professionals in Christian counseling, he has reminded Christian counselors of the profound importance of the Word of God.

The third category is the *Christian Professional*. These men are Christians who have professional training in psychiatry or psychology. Many (Narramore, Dobson, Thurman, Crabb, Hemfelt, Meier, Collins, Mallory, and Hyder, to name a few) are best known for their writings. Although the books of the authors mentioned above reflect a dominant belief in the final standard of authority of God's Word, some other Christian professionals have relied too heavily upon psychology and not enough upon God's Word.

The fourth category is the *Theoretician-Researcher*. These men have studied and researched the field of theology and psychology as they have attempted to provide an apologetic to face the anti-Christian challenge. Collins pointed out in his paper that Freud (psychoanalytic approach), Skinner (behaviorist), and Rogers (humanistic) have all attacked the very basis of Christianity. The theoretician-researchers feel that Christian counselors should be able to give biblical answers. They also feel scientific data is of much importance when dealing with non-Christians.

The last category is comprised of the *Evangelical Popularizers*. These men usually have little professional training in psychology. However, they have significant insights into helping people in a practical, scriptural way and have become well known across the country. The popular writers and speakers in this group include Bill Gothard, Keith Miller, Tim LaHaye, and Bill Gillam.

As can be seen from the above categories, Christian counseling includes several fields: ministers, psychologists, psychiatrists, and related fields. Each needs the other. The minister has the biblical expertise that the others often do not have. The psychologist has the tools for objective evaluations, and the social worker often has special expertise in interpersonal relations. Often, they can greatly benefit a patient by working as a team, whether simultaneously or by referral from one to the other.

The Uniqueness of Christian Counseling

Christian counseling could be defined as the ministry of one individual seeking to help another individual recognize, understand, and solve his own problems in accordance with the Word of God.[43] The emphasis in the above definition is on only two individuals—the patient and the therapist. This emphasis is valid, yet Christian counseling has even further implications. The entire body of Christ in a local area has a responsibility to minister to the emotional needs of one of its members, and the counselor will do well to take advantage in therapy of the tremendous rehabilitative resources (fellowship and spiritual encouragement) available in a local church.

Whether one thinks of the entire local church or the one-to-one relationship when Christian counseling is mentioned and whether the Christian counselor is a minister, psychologist, psychiatrist, or social worker, certain principles make Christian counseling unique.

First, it accepts the Bible as the final standard of authority. As a result, Christians are not left to explore and dissect through the myriad of philosophies and their own logic, and to hope by chance to hit upon a correct system of right and wrong.

What's more, Christians do not have to depend totally upon their own consciences to direct their behavior. They may rely upon the Word of God. If one's conscience agrees with the Word of God, then the conscience is valid; if not, the conscience is invalid. For example, in some cultures, a man might feel guilty for seeing his wife in the nude. Should such a man be told to live up to his conscience? His conscience is too strict and should be reeducated according to the Word of God. As mentioned above, in other cases, an individual may have too little conscience because of poor identity-figures. Thus, he may have developed the attitude that society and others are bad and whatever he does to them is all right. This kind of child develops the feeling that he is OK but others are not OK. In contrast to the former example, this is a case of a too-weak conscience, which also needs reeducating according to the Word of God.

Thus, Christian counseling offers not only practical guidelines through the Bible, but it points to one final standard of authority—the Bible. All schools of thought in psychiatry need a foundation and framework from which to build. The Bible is that foundation for Christian counselors.

The Bible is not primarily a book of rules on rights and wrongs. It is meant to give guidelines, spiritual nourishment, and "life." The Lord Jesus Christ expressed this concept well when He stated, ". . . The words that I speak unto you, they are spirit, and they are life" (John 6:63).

The Bible gives Christian counselors a foundation and a framework. It not only gives insights into human behavior, it puts everything into proper perspective. It tells who man is, where man came from, the purpose of man, and the nature of man. By coupling this tremendous foundation with the scientific facts and observations of psychiatry, the Christian counselor has a good vantage point from which to help individuals solve problems.

Second, Christian counseling is unique because it depends not only on man's willpower to be responsible, but also on God's enabling, indwelling power of the Holy Spirit to conquer man's problems. We do not wish to imply that man has no responsibility for his actions, for he does; yet many Christians choose to act irresponsibly. However, our willingness and attempts to be responsible must be coupled with God's power. Through God's power, man need no longer be a slave to a weak will, his past environment, or social situations. Problems do not disappear when one accepts Christ, but there is a new power to deal with them.

Third, Christian counseling is unique because, even though man does have a basic selfish component, he, if a Christian, has a much stronger godly component. In Romans 7:23, Paul gave the description of an internal battle in an individual not unsimilar to Freud's description of the *id, ego,* and *superego.* The description was that of a good law in the individual mind waging war against an evil law in its "members." As a result, the will was overpowered by the evil law, and only through the Spirit of Christ was victory obtained. Also, only through the Spirit of Christ can real spiritual insights be obtained. Apostle Paul stated, "But the natural man [interpreted "psychological man" from the Greek] receiveth not the things of the Spirit of God: for they are foolishness unto him: neither can he know them, because they are spiritually discerned" (1 Corinthians 2:14).

Fourth, Christian counseling is unique in that it offers an effective way to deal with the past as well as the present. Some of the older schools of thought deal almost exclusively with the past, while some of the newer schools of thought in psychiatry deal mostly with the present. Christian counselors can deal with both. The following two verses point to only a couple of ways that can be tremendously effective in dealing with past guilt or worries: "If we confess our sins, He is faithful and righteous to forgive us our sins and to cleanse us from all unrighteousness" (1 John 1:9 NAS); and ". . . one thing I do: forgetting what *lies* behind and reaching forward to what *lies* ahead. I press on . . ." (Philippians 3:13, 14 NAS). Of course, the counselor cannot always expect a patient to get well by simply pointing out these verses; he must work with each person individually as he helps the person gain insight and victory over his problems.

The fifth reason Christian counseling is unique is that it is based on God's love. Apostle John stated, "In this is love, not that we loved God, but that He loved us and sent His Son to be the propitiation for our sins" (1 John 4:10 NAS). Because God loved us, and His love flows through us, we love others and feel a responsibility toward them. Again, Apostle John states, ". . . whoever loves the Father loves the *child* born of Him" (1 John

5:1 NAS). The Christian counselor feels a spiritual relationship with other Christians and hopes to help them grow in Christ as they solve their problems. The Christian counselor hopes the non-Christian accepts the Lord. Christ died for this individual, and his first step to finding real inner peace is through knowing Christ.

The sixth reason Christian counseling is unique is that it is universal. It can apply to all people regardless of genetic, social, educational, or cultural background. The psychoanalytic school, the transactional analysts, the reality therapists, all recognize that there are certain types of people they can help better than others. Christ claimed He could help all who would turn to Him (*see* Matthew 11:28; John 6:37). Of course, this does not mean that Christian counselors can help all people, but that Christ forms the foundation of their counseling, and He can help all who are willing to turn to Him.

The last reason Christian counseling is unique is that it truly seeks to deal with the whole person. The Christian counselor knows that the physical, psychological, and spiritual aspects of man are all intricately related, and that when one aspect is affected, the other two are also. For example, an ulcer may start on a physical level. Some individuals have a defect in their stomach lining and are thus predisposed to ulcers. Then perhaps because of factors in an individual's upbringing laid down early in life, he or she may be prone to be a very serious person, plagued by fears and worry, which worsens the ulcer. Finally, some spiritual crisis occurs that relates to an area of chosen sin or possibly an issue of deep doubt that drives a wedge between the individual and his relationship with his Creator. The result may first surface physically as a bleeding ulcer. Physical, psychological, and spiritual factors have now all combined to form the presenting problem facing the counselor.

In another case, perhaps the problem did not start on a physical or psychological level, but on a spiritual level. For example, the individual may have chosen to sin and commit adultery. His guilt feelings may lead to anxiety and then to an ulcer or some other physiologic problem.

In summary, man is very intricate in his makeup, and usually when one aspect of man is affected, so are the other parts.

We would take issue with those who either deny the spiritual aspect or deny the psychological aspect. Considering the objective data available today, it is clear that psychological problems exist, and certainly not all of them are directly related to spiritual factors. For example, children deprived of love in the first few weeks of life will develop severe depression and may even die. Is this a spiritual problem at this age?

Not treating the whole man is tragic because of the limitations the counselor imposes upon himself when he denies the reality of the other dimensions of man. For example, can one imagine treating a diabetic with spiritual exhortation? In like manner, treating a person with biochemical depression with spiritual exhortation alone can result in much anguish for the counselee. And how could one treat *anaclitic depression* (a psychological problem) in a baby with a spiritual approach alone? Finally, how can a counselor treat a spiritual problem if he uses only psychological and physical therapies? *Man is a whole, composed of more than one part, and he must be treated as such.*

To determine whether a problem started on a physical, psychological, or spiritual level, each level should be evaluated. A counselee with any evidence of a physical problem should be referred to a physician for a complete physical evaluation. A check into the spiritual aspect should also be done and include such questions as: Does the patient need to know Christ? Is he spiritually immature and in need of growing in Christ? Would he thus benefit from a plan for Scripture memory or Bible study? Is there a specific sin he needs to face? Finally, in some cases, initial attention should be given to the psychological aspect. For example, does the counselee have what used to be called a "neurosis" (cannot function adequately biologically or socially), a *psychosis* (a loss of contact with reality), a *psychophysiologic disorder* (ulcer, colitis, etc.), or a personality disorder? In the above cases, a medical doctor and a minister may need to work together. Again, the parts are integrally related and the counselor needs to recognize and deal with all three parts and their interrelations. *Man is a whole and must be dealt with as such.*

The Balance Needed in Christian Counseling

Just as balance is the key to both spiritual and emotional maturity, so is balance the key to successful Christian counseling. For example, Jesus Christ Himself had tremendous balance. He knew when to be directive and when to help others gain insight through parables (*see* John 2). He knew when to focus on the present without excluding the past (*see* John 4). He knew when to focus on the spiritual aspect of man but not neglect the physical and psychological aspects (*see* John 5).

The Apostle Paul also had emotional and spiritual balance. In 1 Thessalonians 5:14, Paul recorded the balance that is needed in counseling. I first noted this verse while I was in my residency training in psychiatry. As I was studying one day and attempting to integrate my newly found psychiatric knowledge with Scripture, my eyes fell on this verse:

> And we urge you, brethren, admonish the unruly, encourage the fainthearted, help the weak, be patient with all men.
>
> 1 THESSALONIANS 5:14 NAS

As we read the verse, we note that everyone was not counseled in the same manner. Some were admonished, or in present-day terminology, they were treated with a matter-of-fact approach. Some were encouraged, an approach that makes us think of a psychiatric approach known as "active friendliness." And yet, others were to be helped in a supportive, friendly manner. *All* were to be treated with patience.

Thus, psychiatrically and biblically, it becomes evident that everyone should not be counseled in the same way. At times, a counselor should be confronting, at other times not; an active, friendly approach would help some individuals, while others would only become worse with this approach. In short, one type of counseling would not work with all individuals.

Certainly the Scriptures are the basis for the truths in counseling, but the personal application of these truths will vary with the particular need of the counselee. It is part of the role of the effective counselor to know when to be "gentle as a lamb, or shrewd as a serpent" in his or her approach.

Aspects of Biblical Counseling

There are five variations of biblical verbs on counseling. They are: *parakaleo, noutheteo, parmutheomai, antechomai,* and *makrothumeo.*[44, 45]

These five Greek verbs are used in 1 Thessalonians 5:14 mentioned above. The first is *parakaleo.* Paul used this counseling verb himself as he began his statement on the different types of counseling. It means to beseech or exhort, encourage or comfort. It is used in a milder sense than the next verb, which means to admonish. In the original Greek text, this next verb is found in Romans 12:1, 2 Corinthians 1:4, and Romans 15:30 quoted respectively below:

> I beseech you therefore, brethren, by the mercies of God, that ye present your bodies a living sacrifice, holy, acceptable unto God, which is your reasonable service.
>
> ROMANS 12:1

> Who comforteth us in all our tribulation, that we may be able to comfort them which are in any trouble, by the comfort wherewith we ourselves are comforted of God.
>
> 2 CORINTHIANS 1:4

> Now I beseech you, brethren, for the Lord Jesus Christ's sake, and for the love of the Spirit, that ye strive together with me in your prayers to God for me.
>
> ROMANS 15:30

It is an active verb. It is the verb on which Paul Morris bases his counseling known as "Love Therapy."

The next Greek verb is *noutheteo.* This verb can be used in a broad context in counseling, but in the New Testament it usually means to put in mind, to warn, and to confront. It is intended to produce a change in life-style. One especially admonishes the unruly, the undisciplined, or the impulsive, but we also admonish one another. It is found in the verses quoted on the next page:

And concerning you, my brethren, I myself also am convinced
that you yourselves are full of goodness, filled with all knowledge,
and able also to admonish one another.

ROMANS 15:14 NAS

I am not writing this to shame you, but to warn you, as my dear
children.

1 CORINTHIANS 4:14 NIV

Let the word of Christ richly dwell within you, with all wisdom
teaching and admonishing one another with psalms *and* hymns
and spiritual songs, singing with thankfulness in your hearts to
God.

1 COLOSSIANS 3:16 NAS

It is also an active verb. It is the verb on which Jay Adams
bases his Nouthetic Counseling.

The third counseling verb is *parmutheomai.* It means to have
a positive attitude, to cheer up, to encourage. One encourages
the fainthearted or discouraged. It is found in the original Greek
text as follows:

Just as you know how we *were* exhorting and encouraging and
imploring each one of you as a father *would* his own children.

1 THESSALONIANS 2:11 NAS

The fourth counseling verb is *antechomai.* It means to be
available, to cling to, to hold fast, to take an interest in, to hold
up spiritually or emotionally. It is a passive verb.

The fifth Greek verb is *makrothumeo.* It means to be patient
or to have persistence. It is found in Matthew 18:26, Matthew
18:29, James 5:7, and Hebrews 6:15. It is also a passive verb.

Thus, there is not just one biblical verb on counseling, but
there are several, a fact which proves that a person needs balance in his counseling approach. Christian counseling is *unique*
in its ability to provide this balance.

I do not frustrate the grace of God:
for if righteousness come by the law,
then Christ is dead in vain.

GALATIANS 2:21

2 The Theology of Healthy Christian Counseling (Grace vs. a Double-Bind Message)

The Damage of a Double-Bind Message

Untold psychological damage is done when an individual feels he is accepted by ones that are close to him only on a conditional basis. This may be expressed in a contradictory message, such as verbally relating, "I love you," but in actions relating, "If you want me to continue to love you, you must. . . ."

Similar to a contradictory message, but even more damaging, is a message known as a *double-bind*. This message produces a paradox that makes choice impossible. With a double-bind message, a child is asked to do two conflicting things. He may be verbally asked to be good, but the covert message is to "act out." If the child is bad, he violates the verbal message asking him to be good. However, if he is good, he violates the covert message asking him to "act out." He cannot win. Whatever decision he makes, he loses.

Although a double-bind message such as the one above can be very detrimental to a child and even contributes to the loss of contact with reality known as *schizophrenia*, an even more serious *double-bind* message is given from many pulpits every Sunday. When a minister asks someone to do something for the grace of God, he has just given the individual an impossible choice. By definition, grace is God's unmerited favor. It cannot

33

be earned, for this would contradict the definition. Thus, if the individual chooses grace, he cannot do anything for it. Yet, the minister has told him something he must do. The individual cannot win under this system. He is under a *double-bind* message.

An understanding of the concept of grace is basic to the prevention of a double-bind message being given from a pulpit. What follows is a development of that concept, a concept that is basic to both the Bible and psychiatry.

Grace as a Foundation for Christian Psychiatry

Grace is a concept which so easily escapes us. Indeed, it is a concept foreign to the way of life of most humans and thus hard to appreciate. Because of our psychological makeup, man through the centuries has repeatedly gravitated from the concept of grace to that of law.[1]

Men like Martin Luther stand as stalwarts in Christian history as men who once again discovered the marvelous meaning of grace. After years of striving in vain to be righteous, and after years of psychological pain, Martin Luther found a solution for the basic guilt common to man. This was the beginning of the Protestant Reformation, and the world had little known such widespread joy since the early Church.

How the Church views grace has widespread implications. A misconception in one direction results in depression, while a misconception in another direction results in a perceived "license to sin." A misconception of the term "grace" carries not only widespread spiritual implications, but also psychological harm.

Raising Healthy Children—An Example of Grace in Action

God gave us the example of how to produce healthy children when He chose that the foundation of a relationship between two individuals should be based on the concept of grace. Grace implies that the love of God is free and unmerited. Just as parents usually accept their children and will have an innate love for them regardless of what they do, so God loves us. Although God does not always like our behavior, just as parents do not always like their children's behavior, there is a great difference between not accepting someone's behavior and not accepting that person. Children still feel loved if parents do not accept their irresponsible behavior, but they feel rejected and discouraged if they feel that they themselves are rejected. This type of rejection leads to discouragement, neurosis, and even psychosis. Likewise, Christians may become discouraged, neurotic, or even psychotic if they feel their receiving or keeping Christ is conditional.

In some teaching today, it is tragic that God's system of grace has been mongrelized into a *grace-plus-merit* system. Consequently, rather than receiving Christ's unconditional love and giving of ourselves as a result, some teachers encourage others to merely give their lives to Christ. God has already condemned the old sin, nature, and made atonement on the Cross. He does not want one to *give* but to *receive.* Evangelical sermons too often put the emphasis on what one is to *do*—commitments, public confessions, restitution, etc.—rather than on receiving and living as an expression of the love and devotion that Christ demonstrated on the Cross.

Grace Versus Debt, Works, Law

Grace is set in contrast to debt, works, and law in Scripture.[2] *The American College Dictionary* defines these terms in some of the important details listed below.[3] In Romans 4:4, grace is set in contrast with debt. Debt implies that one owes another and must pay or perform for that debt. It implies an obligation. Theologically, it implies that an offense has been committed and requires reparation. In leading others to Christ, an emphasis on a performance of some kind, an obligation, or reparation is an emphasis on debt, which God sets in contrast to grace.

Second, grace is set in contrast to works in Romans 11:6. Work refers to the result of labor or activity. It refers to a deed or a performance. Theologically, it refers to an act of obedience. Work refers to obtaining something by effort. A synonym for work is "toil," which is wearying and exhausting. Thus, in leading others to Christ, an emphasis on an action in response to obedience, on exertion that takes much willpower and is exhausting, or any other labor is an emphasis on works, which is in contrast to God's concept of grace (*see* Ephesians 2:8, 9; Titus 3:5).

Third, grace is set in contrast to law in Galatians 5:4 and in John 1:17. A law implies a regulation that should be kept. I have heard Christian workers say, "I like to tell someone about the Christian life before he becomes a Christian, so he will know what to expect." Their aim is to obtain from the person a resolution to live the Christian life. However, a Christian worker putting emphasis on resolutions is in contrast with God and His emphasis on grace.

The power to live the Christian life is given by the indwelling power of the Holy Spirit that comes at the time one receives Christ. Without this power, all actions are based on *willpower* (human), which God condemns (*see* John 1:13). God gives grace to a non-Christian to understand the plan of God in salvation and then to accept Christ, resulting in a change of attitude about himself, sin, and Christ; but beyond this, the Holy Spirit must produce results.

We evangelical Christians consent to the concept of grace versus law. However, we, too, if not careful, will be prone to a tendency to progress from grace to a mixed *grace-merit* system. This results because the idea of grace as unmerited favor is largely foreign to our society and also to our way of thinking.

A Psychiatric Example—The Unpardonable Sin

An endless frustration or perhaps, even worse, a temporary soothing of the conscience is produced by a *grace-plus-merit* system. Dr. Minirth's treatment of a recent patient at the clinic illustrates this principle well. This patient was a college girl with whom he had been working for two to three weeks with little progress. She had been admitted to the hospital for an overdose of sedative pills that she had taken because of depression. Efforts were made repeatedly to gain rapport and encourage her to talk but had largely failed. She remained inwardly angry and hostile. She admitted there was something about which she was unwilling to talk and had given the staff some insight into her problem on the night of her admission to the hospital. She asked if a person had to walk to the front of the church to be saved. She was assured then that one did not. She stated that she agreed, but that she knew many people who would disagree with the view that a person need do nothing more than accept Jesus Christ as his Savior to establish the right relationship with God. Was the advice offered too quickly rather than initially listening more? Therapy then progressed slowly after her admission to the hospital until one session three weeks later. The patient had some things on her conscience she really needed to share. Dr. Minirth thus began to ask her questions that would enable her to share her stressful burden:

> I asked, "When did it occur?"
>
> She stated, "At the age of sixteen." She later explained that what she had done would make others think she was terrible, and that it was the most horrible thing anyone could do. Finally, I confined the problem to an issue between her and God. She felt she had committed the unpardonable sin.
>
> I asked, "What do you think the unpardonable sin is? Individuals think differently. What do you think it is?"
>
> I then proceeded to share with her some thoughts others have had about the unpardonable sin (*see* Mark 3:28, Matthew 12:31, and Luke 12:10). An unpardonable sin would be the rejection of the Holy Spirit for the last time after which a person would never be convicted again. Of course, after death, grace would no longer be offered, and the sin of unbelief would no longer be pardonable. I shared with her that the very fact that she wanted to know Christ meant that she had not committed the unpardonable sin.
>
> The other concept of an unpardonable sin would be equating the Holy Spirit with evil. This would be a matter of the heart, as when the scribes stated Christ performed his miracles by the power of Satan.
>
> She thought there was still perhaps another way she had committed the unpardonable sin, and that was by attending a worship service of the devil with a friend of hers who claimed to be a witch. I shared with her the thought that I could not recall one verse of Scripture that would deem this unpardonable.

Another proof that she had not committed the unpardonable sin would be if she were a Christian. However, she was unsure at this point, and I asked, "Have you ever invited Christ into your life?"

She answered, "Yes, many times."

Later, I had the opportunity to read a note she had written as a rather young girl which read something like this: "My friends ask me if I am a Christian. I answer 'yes,' but to me my being a Christian is different from *their* being Christians. To me being a Christian is between me and Christ, but to them, it is between them and other people. To them, being a Christian is telling other people, but to me it is telling Christ. . . ."

I was impressed with the depth and spiritual wisdom of her thinking as a little child. Apparently, she had become a Christian at an early age, but then with further exposure to the *grace-plus-merit* system, combined with her own *obsessive-compulsive* personality trends, she succumbed to guilt and frustration.

She stated, "I am going to hell. I just know it."

I asked, "How do you know it?"

She answered, "Because I have not done enough right."

I asked, "Do you know what God thinks of our righteousness? He thinks 'our righteousnesses are as filthy rags . . .' (*see* Isaiah 64:6). So do you know what we get if we try to get to heaven by the *right* things we do? We get a debt rather than heaven."

I then asked her to visualize Christ on the Cross, to visualize all her sins, to then visualize each sin driving a spike into His hand, and finally to visualize carrying all her guilt up to the Cross and giving it to Christ. She had an anguished demeanor.

I asked, "Can you visualize what I have said?"

"Yes," was the answer.

I proceeded, "Visualize Christ standing at your heart's door and knocking, and then visualize yourself opening the door and asking Him to come into your life."

I then shared John 6:37: "All that the Father giveth me shall come to me; and him that cometh to me, I will in no wise cast out."

I repeated the quote and then shared Ephesians 2:8, 9: "For by grace are ye saved through faith; and that not of yourselves: it is the gift of God: Not of works, lest any man should boast."

I repeated this also and stated, "Nothing to boast about. If I could do something, I could boast; but I can't."

Soon a serene, peaceful look came over the patient's face "Is the guilt gone?" I asked.

"Yes," was the response

The patient then slowly began to improve despite her problems. Although this patient would not instantly be free of psychological problems, I was glad I had the opportunity to introduce her to grace.

What we *do* and *don't do* in the Christian life is not based on a brownie-point system, but on a love for Christ and a respect for His wisdom. He is so much wiser than we, that we would be foolish not to follow his leading. In Isaiah 55:8, 9, God recorded, "For my thoughts are not your thoughts, neither are your ways my ways, saith the Lord. For as the heavens are higher than the earth, so are my ways higher than your ways, and my thoughts than your thoughts." Jeremiah 29:11 reflects God's general attitude when He said to Israel, "For I know the thoughts that I think toward you, saith the Lord, thoughts of peace, and not of evil, to give you an expected end."

The Simplicity of Christ

In 2 Corinthians 11:3, 4, Apostle Paul referred to the fear he had that the Corinthians might be led astray from the simplicity and purity of devotion to Christ, and that they might be corrupted with another (different) gospel. The idea of another gospel is again mentioned in Galatians. The Gospel is very simply the good news that Jesus Christ the Son of God died on the Cross in payment for man's sins, and that He not only died but rose from the grave after three days and had victory over sin and death. This is payment in full to God and nothing one can do can add to this. This is grace. Others have written excellent in-depth books on the subject, and just the general concepts of grace will be reviewed here.[4–11]

Grace says, "Believe only."

Law says, "Believe plus do something."

Grace says, "Everything has been accomplished for your salvation; now only receive."
Law says, "You must do in order to receive."

Grace says, "All has been accomplished; now rest."
Law says, "You owe a debt."

Grace says, "Receive Christ as Savior, and then do."
Grace says, "Salvation is based on Christ's merit and on our
believing."
Law says, "Salvation is based, at least to some degree, on human merit."

Law requires various works for salvation: a good life, dedica-
tion, vows, resolutions, commitments, prayer, public confession, charity, and baptism. But it is the Holy Spirit who enables
Christians "both to will and to do of his good pleasure" (*see*
Philippians 2:13).

The list of examples could be continued, and one must remember that some *grace-plus-work* systems are much more subtle in their approaches than others. However, the scriptural fact
remains, and is presented repeatedly, that the one condition for
salvation is *belief.*

We should also mention that repentance does occur simultaneously with belief. Repentance literally means a change of attitude with respect to sin, self, and Christ; and this occurs as one
turns away from self to Christ for salvation. Finally, belief is
more than intellectual consent; belief involves a relationship
with Christ; i.e., bowing our will to His preeminence.

Just as the Christian life is started in the Spirit by faith, so it
is lived that way. The life we are called to live under the principles of grace is a much higher standard than could ever be
imposed by the law, because under grace and in Christ, we have
the enabling power of the Holy Spirit working through us.

Reasons for Legalism

At this point, the question may arise as to why we are prone
to becoming legalistic or imposing legalistic standards on others.
Four apparent reasons come to mind. The first is ignorance. If

we have heard of grace-plus or heard of grace with some human obligation added, this may have programmed our minds toward difficulty in understanding true grace. In addition, if we ignorantly view God as human beings tend to do, we will have difficulty understanding unmerited favor.

Second, guilt and a psychiatric concept of reaction formation alluded to previously may be important. Reaction formations may be healthy or unhealthy. If the reaction results in a person's becoming legalistic with others because he really wants to live a loose moral life, this is unhealthy. One counselee was a minister and hated hypocrisy in the church. He little realized, until later in therapy, that he was very much a hypocrite himself and was probably practicing his ministry as a result of guilt, compensation, and reaction formation.

Third, well-meaning individuals in their zeal may become legalistic (*see* Romans 10:2). Finally, people become legalistic for their own glory and selfish recognition (*see* Galatians 6:12, 13).

Christ in Us

Verses that deal with the importance of our dependence upon Christ as we cooperate with His revealed Word in Scripture are:

Zechariah 4:6, ". . . Not by might, nor by power, but by my spirit, saith the Lord of hosts."

John 15:5, "I am the vine, ye are the branches: He that abideth in me, and I in him, the same bringeth forth much fruit: for without me ye can do nothing."

Galatians 2:20, 21, "I am crucified with Christ: nevertheless, I live; yet not I, but Christ liveth in me: and the life which I now live in the flesh I live by the faith of the Son of God, who loved me and gave himself for me. I do not frustrate the grace of God: for if righteousness come by the law, then Christ is dead in vain."

Romans 1:17, "For therein is the righteousness of God revealed from faith to faith: as it is written, The just shall live by faith."

GRACE	vs.	LAW
Salvation is a gift (Ephesians 2:8, 9)		Salvation requires a payment by the individual
Demerit cannot result in salvation being denied (Romans 5:8)		Demerit can result in denial of salvation
Personal merit cannot result in salvation being given (Galatians 5:6)		Personal merit can result in salvation
Grace plus nothing (Galatians 4:9)		Grace plus merit
Starts with what Christ has done (Hebrews 7:16)		Starts with what individual must do
Only believe (in Gospels over 115 times)		Believe plus . . .
Receive and then do . . .		Do to receive
Contrasted to a. debt (Romans 4:4, 10) b. works (Romans 11:6) c. law (Galatians 5:14)		Consistent with debt, works, and law

Questions on Grace

Galatians is a book in the New Testament written by the Apostle Paul because the church at Galatia had evolved from a grace to a *grace-plus-merit* system. Paul makes several significant points concerning grace.

1. Is it possible to just trust in Christ, and then find one is not really a Christian?
No, this is not possible (*see* Galatians 2:18).

2. What is the result of combining faith with some other merit?
One sins when he combines faith with personal merit (*see* Galatians 2:18).

3. Who enables the Christian to obey God?

Christ, not the law, enables the Christian to obey God (*see* Galatians 2:20, 21).

4. What happens if one feels obligated to earn salvation and does not feel Christ's righteousness is enough?

He frustrates the grace of God (*see* Galatians 2:21).

5. What does God say about those who present a *grace-plus* system for salvation?

He says they mislead others, hinder them, and actually keep them from obeying the truth rather than obeying it (*see* Galatians 3:1). This persuasion is not from God (*see* Galatians 5:7).

6. Does God consider one wise or foolish who combines grace with merit?

He considers him foolish (*see* Galatians 3:3).

7. Can law (personal merit) and faith coexist?

No, they cannot coexist (*see* Galatians 3:12, 18).

8. Since we are under grace, can anything be added to the condition for salvation?

No, nothing can be added to the one requirement for salvation, and that requirement is faith in Christ (*see* Galatians 3:24).

9. Did the law have a useful purpose?

Yes, the law did have a useful purpose (*see* Galatians 3:19). It still is useful in that it shows the non-Christian that he has sinned and cannot keep the law and thus needs Christ.

10. Is it possible for the *grace-plus-merit* system to give life and peace?

No, this system cannot give life and peace (*see* Galatians 4:9).

11. How does a person feel who is in a *grace-plus-merit* system?

He feels in bondage (*see* Galatians 4:9).

12. What does God command that Christians do in regard to a *grace-plus-merit* system?

Cast it out (*see* Galatians 4:30).

13. If a person is to be justified by personal merit, what must he do?

Keep the whole law, never sin (*see* Galatians 5:3).

14. Do ordinances avail anything in salvation?

No, they avail nothing (*see* Galatians 5:6; Ephesians 2:15).

15. What does personal merit (commitments, confessions, ordinances, restitution) result in if done for salvation?

It results in personal glory (*see* Galatians 6:14).

16. Why can one not earn salvation in just any way?

Because by definition it is a gift, and by definition, a gift is free and belongs to the recipient upon receiving it (*see* Ephesians 2:8, 9).

17. Where do good works fit into God's plan?

They are a result of salvation (*see* Ephesians 2:10).

18. Is it possible for a person to "fall from grace"?

No, one cannot fall from grace (*see* Romans 11:29). According to this verse, God never takes away a gift He has given and eternal life is defined as a gift (*see* Romans 6:23).

19. Why is it a *double-bind* message to combine grace with merit?

By definition, grace is God's unmerited favor. By definition, a gift (eternal life mentioned in Romans 6:23) is free. This means that one cannot earn grace because this would contradict the definition. Thus, when a minister asks someone to do something for the grace of God, he has just presented the individual with an impossible choice. If the individual chooses grace, he cannot do anything for it. Yet, the minister has told him that he must do something. The individual cannot win under this system. He is under a *double-bind* message

The Apostle Paul wrote about aspects of this *double-bind* message; a message that would purport we are righteous by faith, yet somehow need to be justified by works.

> What then shall we say that Abraham, our forefather, discovered in this matter? If, in fact, Abraham was justified by works, he had something to boast about—but not before God. What does the Scripture say? "Abraham believed God, and it was credited to him as righteousness."
>
> Now when a man works, his wages are not credited to him as a gift, but as an obligation. However, to the man who does not work but trusts God who justifies the wicked, his faith is credited as righteousness. David says the same thing when he speaks of the blessedness of the man to whom God credits righteousness apart from works:
>
> "Blessed are they whose transgressions are forgiven, whose sins are covered.
>
> "Blessed is the man whose sin the Lord will never count against him."
>
> ROMANS 4:1–8 NIV

20. Is the individual who ascribes to law or the one who ascribes to grace the healthier mentally?

The one under grace is healthier mentally. In fact, legalism can produce serious spiritual and psychological problems. The author of Hebrews wrote that it was good for the heart to be established by grace (*see* Hebrews 13:9)

Grace—A Foundation for Biblical Teaching and Christian Psychiatry

When one becomes a Christian, he chooses with his will to believe in Christ. He does not necessarily need nor is he required to will a commitment beyond this, though he may. But to require a commitment beyond this is to require more than God requires.

One may pull verses out of context in the Bible and prove anything he wishes. By this, he can prove that public confession, baptism, restitution, strong commitments, and good works are all necessary to salvation. By this method, he can prove that salvation can be denied because of demerits and past sins. Although men do this, when considering any work, the whole theme should be considered. The whole theme of the Bible is *grace*. The whole plot builds toward this end and is directed at this.

In psychiatry, a foundation of therapy is that the patient feels the therapist accepts him (but not his irresponsible behavior) unconditionally. To be sure, this is the same foundation God chose for His relationship to man. To this end, Chafer, Nee, Scofield, Luther, and Spurgeon wrote about the unconditional grace of God. We personally believe this principle needs reemphasizing today. An understanding of grace is foundational to Christian psychiatry as well as to the Bible.

> . . . I pray God your whole spirit and
> soul and body be preserved blame-
> less unto the coming of our Lord
> Jesus Christ.
>
> 1 THESSALONIANS 5:23

3 A Comparison of Christian Psychiatry, Psychoanalysis, and Transactional Analysis

Psychiatry's Main Thrust

Psychiatry's major thrust has been helping an individual make appropriate changes in his soul (mind, will, and emotions) that will enable him to overcome or cope with his particular problem. For instance, psychoanalysis has dealt primarily with the subconscious (one component of the mind), as well as helping the patient understand his feelings (a function of the emotions). Transactional analysis, on the contrary, has focused on a different aspect of the mind (the logical, rational, mature, thinking aspect) and has also placed strong emphasis on the will, stating that we can determine our course in life and conquer our problems.

The Rationale Behind the Thrust

What is the rationale behind the particular thrusts of the different therapies within the field of psychotherapy or counseling? The thrust to a large extent depends upon the particular concept of the parts of man. Just what makes up a human being? The parts, and the struggle between the parts resulting in emotional conflict, are constituents of the psychoanalytic theory, the description in transactional analysis, and the description in the Bible.

Psychoanalytic Theory and the Parts of Man

The psychoanalytic theory holds that the important parts of man are the *superego, id,* and *ego.* These terms have become famous and are in common usage in both secular and religious settings. According to this theory, the *superego* is the conscience. The *id* represents the basic drives, such as those for food and sex. The *ego* has the responsibility of weighing between the pressures of the id and those of the superego, thus acting as the logical, rational, objective, reality-oriented decision-maker. Anxiety may occur as a result of striving between these internal parts of man. Consider the following diagram:

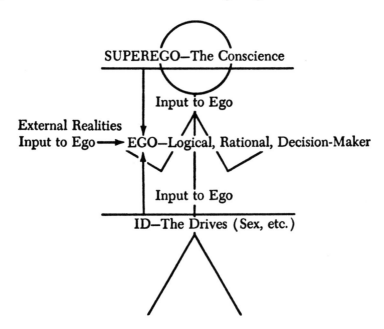

Transactional Analysis and the Parts of Man

A counselor in transactional analysis holds that man consists of a parent, child, and an adult. The "parent" judges, the "child" emphasizes his feelings, and the "adult" acts logically and in a rational manner. In transactions with others, we are always acting and feeling like one of these entities. Consider the following diagram:

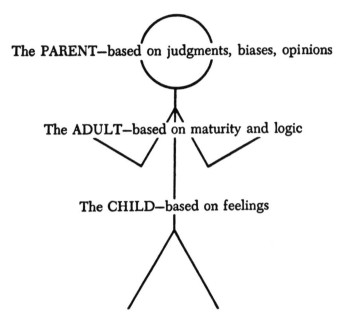

The PARENT—based on judgments, biases, opinions

The ADULT—based on maturity and logic

The CHILD—based on feelings

The Bible Contrasted with Secular Theory

The Bible, too, speaks of the importance of the parts of man. There is a good and strikingly close correlation between the description given in the Bible and that formulated from observations and theories in psychiatry. However, there are differences. The Bible and secular theorists are alike in that they describe the struggles between the parts of man. For example, psychoanalysis describes a struggle between the drives in man (*id*) and his conscience (*superego*). The will must consider both and also reality and choose what to do. The Bible describes the struggle between carnal desires and the Holy Spirit in a Christian. However, the descriptions are different in that one is a theory and pertains to man without Christ, and the other is a fact and pertains to the Christian.

One cannot equate the Spirit in the Christian with the conscience in the psychoanalytic system because a non-Christian's conscience results mainly from early parental teachings. In a Christian, the Holy Spirit is also a major influence in the conscience. Consider the diagrams below:

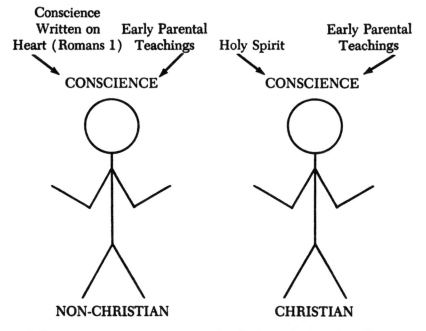

Likewise, one cannot equate the flesh with the *id* in the psychoanalytic system because the *id* by definition contains all drives. Drives can be expressed in inappropriate or evil ways, but drives in and of themselves are not evil.

Because of similar arguments, one cannot say that the parent, adult, and child of transactional analysis are parts of the soul. We would say, although most transactional analysts would heartily disagree, that the parent, adult, and child of transactional analysis are similar to the *superego, ego,* and *id* of psychoanalysis. In the diagram on the next page, similarities of the systems are noted.

The thrust of therapy may differ because of the importance relegated to each particular part. For example, in the past, psychoanalysis has viewed neurosis, at times, as resulting from the inhibitions of the *id*'s drive for sexual aggression. Thus, in this conceptual framework, the superego might be viewed as patho-

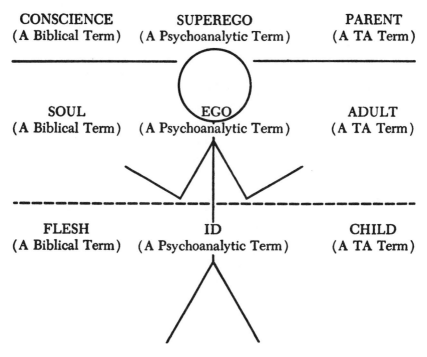

| CONSCIENCE | SUPEREGO | PARENT |
| (A Biblical Term) | (A Psychoanalytic Term) | (A TA Term) |

| SOUL | EGO | ADULT |
| (A Biblical Term) | (A Psychoanalytic Term) | (A TA Term) |

| FLESH | ID | CHILD |
| (A Biblical Term) | (A Psychoanalytic Term) | (A TA Term) |

logical, and therapy thus directed may be viewed as weakening the conscience. The transactional analysis, on the other hand, places much importance on the concept of the adult in each of us. Here the thrust of therapy is on the will. Likewise, the Bible speaks to the parts of man. It considers man in a whole conceptual framework. Furthermore, the thrust is on an aspect of man that psychiatry has tried in vain to avoid, namely, the spiritual.

Psychiatry has tried to sidestep the spiritual aspect of man. The secular views of the parts of man are not so erroneous as they are incomplete. They are ignorant of the spiritual aspect of man. Logically, the idea of relating to others as an adult, parent, or child at any given time is reasonable. In fact, it seems quite simple. And the psychoanalytic concepts of a conscience (*super-ego*), drives (*id*), and logic (*ego*) do not seem more than common sense. These secular views of the parts of man are just incomplete. As a medical doctor, the psychiatrist pays attention to any physical problems. Likewise, he is very concerned with the patient's mind, emotions, and will. He desires to give the patient stability in these areas. Yet, even if all parts of man were equal, the traditional psychiatrist has ignored a third aspect of man. He has ignored the spiritual aspect. *How can a third of the whole be ignored?* Can denial be used to ignore a part of man on the assumption that it should not be dealt with by the counselor? Can man be fractionated and each part dealt with separately?

Theologians have long debated whether man is dichotomous (consisting of two parts) or trichotomous (consisting of three parts). Personally, we feel the trichotomy theory is accurate. Others have written extensively about these parts, but the following is a brief review.[1-8]

Man desires to be dealt with as a whole. The Bible describes the whole man as consisting of a body, soul, and spirit. Furthermore, it describes in detail the parts of these entities. The Bible's account of the parts of man is the most accurate ever given. It is not based on theory or even sound observation, but on facts. It is based on the words of the One who made man—God Himself. An understanding of these parts of man is basic to sound counseling. Confusion of the functions of one part with functions of another has resulted in much misunderstanding through the years.

Greek and Hebrew Meanings

Man consists of a body, soul, and spirit. In 1 Thessalonians 5:23 (NAS), the following is recorded: "Now may the God of peace Himself sanctify you entirely; and may your spirit and soul and body be preserved complete, without blame at the coming of our Lord Jesus Christ." This is a very significant verse, for it refers to three distinct and separate parts of man. The distinction is not unlike that heard in secular areas where man in totality is referred to as spirit, soul, and body. The reference is to the spiritual aspect of man, the psychological aspect of man, and, finally, the physical aspect. In the above verse, each part is considered separately and each has different functions; yet, they must complement to make a whole. The whole of man is again described in a very early portion of Scripture. In Genesis 2:7 NAS, the following is recorded: "Then the Lord God formed man of dust from the ground [Hebrew word for body is *basar*], and breathed into his nostrils the breath of life [Hebrew word *neshamah*, meaning the human spirit, is used here]; and man became a living being [can also be translated "soul"—Hebrew word for soul here is *nephesh*]." Thus, God combined body plus spirit to form the soul. Consider the diagram below.

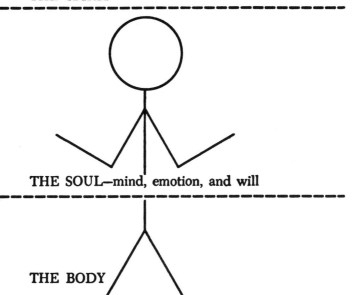

Soul or Psyche

The Greek word for soul is *psyche*. It has various meanings in the New Testament and theologians Chafer, Hodge, Vine, Nee, and Strong differ on whether it should be considered a different entity from spirit. However, we prefer to consider it as separate because of Apostle Paul's statement in 1 Thessalonians 5 quoted on the preceding page (*see* also Hebrews 4:12), and also because from a psychological view this division makes sense. It explains why Christians have emotional problems. This will be discussed later in more detail. Notwithstanding, the word *soul* is most often used as a synonym for the person—the self. In fact, translators have often translated the word *soul* as "self." Hence, Matthew 16:26 and Luke 9:25 have very similar wording but one passage records the word *soul* and the other records the word *self.* Thus, the soul is the *self*—the person. An individual composed of spiritual capacities, plus genetic potentials, results in a unique personality, *self* or *soul.* With his body, man is in contact with the physical world around him. With his spirit, man has the potential of being in contact with the inner or spiritual. In between the two, resides the soul, with its psychological and mental functions.

The Soul—The Psychological

The soul is the psychological aspect of man, whereas the spirit is the spiritual. Psychiatrists and psychologists have focused the thrust of their endeavors at this aspect of man. The hope has been to help individuals with confused minds, weak wills, and labile emotions. The Bible focuses on these three functions of the soul. In Job 7:15 and Job 6:7, reference is made to the ability of the soul to choose (the will). In Proverbs 19:2 and Psalm 139:14, reference is made to the intellectual or knowing aspect of the soul (the mind). Finally, in Song of Solomon 1:7 and 2 Samuel 5:8, reference is made to "emotions" as a function of the soul.

A Christian's problems may be manifested through any one of the parts of the soul. He may be very emotional, and these emotions can spring from a purely psychological base rather than a spiritual. Other Christians may become angry easily or develop bitterness quickly. In addition, a Christian's problem may be manifested through his will. He may identify with the Apostle Paul's statement, ". . . I do the very thing I do not wish to do . . ." (Romans 7:16 NAS). Lastly, the Christian's problem may manifest in his intellect—his mind. He may, like the Pharisees, know every "jot and tittle" of the law and yet be miserable. He fails to recognize that the mind alone lies in the psychological aspect of man and not the spiritual.

The soul would be a major area of attack by Satan. For an

immature Christian, Satan might attack through a carnal expression of the body, such as lust-provoking sights that the eyes behold. However, for a more mature Christian, he might focus the temptation a step deeper into the makeup of man and infect his soul—his mind, emotions, or will. Satan throws mental "darts" (*see* Ephesians 6) figuratively, in an attempt to establish obsessions ("strongholds") and delusions ("imaginations") in the mind of a Christian (*see* 2 Corinthians 10). Thus, Christians do have mental problems and a significant percentage of patients we treat are Christians.

The Christian with mental problems may, as the non-Christian, work at a disadvantage to try to handle his problems. If he is depending on his own ability, his own objectivity, or his own logic, he may very well temporarily improve. Yet, he labors at a distinct disadvantage.

The Spirit or Pneuma

This leads to a discussion of the innermost aspect of man—the *spirit*. The *spirit* is the supernatural part of man given by God at birth. It is not to be equated with the Holy Spirit of God, received by Christians at the time of conversion. The term *spirit* is used to denote several functions in the Bible.

Functions of the Spirit

The following are two key functions of the *spirit*. The first is that the *spirit* is the organ for communion with God. Christ stated, "But an hour is coming, and now is, when the true worshipers shall worship the Father in spirit and truth; for such people the Father seeks to be His worshipers" (John 4:23 NAS). This is why an individual can intellectually know all about Christ and yet never have experienced the joy of a personal relationship with Him

At the time an individual comes to recognize that Christ was the Son of God—that He died on the Cross for his sins, that He rose from the grave and thus was victorious over death—forsakes his own futile efforts to be righteous, and accepts the righteousness of God–Jesus Christ, then he becomes a Christian. When a person believes in Christ or receives Him as his Savior, then the Holy Spirit comes to indwell that person, that person's human *spirit* (*see* John 3:6 NAS).

Another important function of the Spirit is perception and insight. This perception comes from deep within and is independent of mental reasoning. In Mark 2:8, an instance is recorded when the scribes were reasoning but Christ was perceiving in His Spirit. What a contrast! How can one determine if an impression is from the Spirit or just from the mind (soul)? One way is through a living knowledge of the Word of God. The following is recorded: "For the word of God is living and active and sharper than any two-edged sword, and piercing as far as the division of soul and spirit, of both joints and marrow, and able to judge the thoughts and intentions of the heart" (Hebrews 4:12 NAS).

The above paragraph is referring to the conscience as one function of the Holy Spirit. However, the Christian should remember that the Holy Spirit only makes up one factor of the conscience in a Christian and not the whole conscience. The other factors contributing to the conscience of the Christian are the early parental teachings that were both mentally healthy and not mentally healthy (either too rigid or not strict enough). When one understands that one of three factors influencing the conscience of the Christian can be unhealthy, he can understand why Christian as well as non-Christian can have psychological problems in his conscience. The Holy Spirit's convictions are never unhealthy; neither are certain aspects of early parental teachings. However, the unhealthy aspects of early parental teachings do produce problems. For example, parents who are extremely strict, dominating, or legalistic produce a child with a conscience that is always condemning him and that he can never please. Of course, the other extreme (parents who are not strict enough) is equally harmful. Consider the diagram on the following page.

Why Christians Have Emotional Problems

The reasons why Christians have emotional problems are many. Genetics, environment, physical health, and stress are all

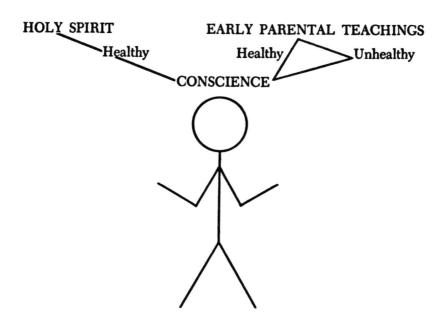

factors. The importance of genetics in personality types and emotional problems is flooding the literature. With studies revealing that children of schizophrenic parents develop schizophrenia even when raised in a healthy home away from their parents, one must be impressed.[9] Likewise, literature has abounded for years with scientific evidence of the importance of environment and stress as factors contributing to emotional problems.

However, there is one factor about the Christian we wish to stress. Many problems could be avoided for the Christian if he just lived a life constantly as Christ wanted him to. He would avoid doing many things that cause guilt, anxiety, and stress. Thus, the following question arises: If Christians have a new life and power within them at the time of conversion, why do they continue to have mental and emotional problems? One reason is that the mind is a part of the soul, not the spirit. The soul does not become new or have any change at the time of conversion; the spirit does. Only after one has spent time in the Word of God, in prayer, and in fellowship, is the mind renewed in accordance with the will of God (*see* Romans 12:1). After receiving Christ, one will sin periodically with vain thoughts and actions because he chooses, unfortunately, to yield his soul to the authority not of the Holy Spirit, as God desires, but rather to the "flesh."

The Sinful Nature of Man—The Sarx

The Greek word for flesh is *sarx*. *Sarx* has a variety of meanings in the New Testament. Among these are: "the source of sin in human nature" (*see* 1 John 2:16); "the weaker element of an individual" (*see* Romans 8:39); and "the carnal element in the Christian" (*see* Galatians 5:17). The Christian may be thrown into a dilemma as both the flesh and the Spirit compete for control. "For the flesh sets its desire against the Spirit, and the Spirit against the flesh; for these are in opposition to one another . . ." (Galatians 5:17 NAS).

Thus, a Christian is very complex in his makeup. Just as psychiatry has surmised, conflict between internal parts can produce anxiety. One of the best examples of the interrelations between the parts of man in producing emotional stress was expressed by Paul:

> For I know that nothing good dwells in me, that is, in my flesh; for the wishing is present in me, but the doing of the good *is* not. For the good that I wish, I do not do; but I practice the very evil that I do not wish. But if I am doing the very thing I do not wish, I am no longer the one doing it, but the sin which dwells in me. I find then the principle that evil is present in me, the one who wishes to do good. For I joyfully concur with the law of God in the inner man, but I see a different law in the members of my body, waging war against the law of my mind, and making me a prisoner of the law of sin which is in my members. Wretched man that I am! Who will set me free from the body of this death? Thanks be to God through Jesus Christ our Lord! So then, on the one hand I myself with my mind am serving the law of God, but on the other, with my flesh the law of sin. There is therefore now no condemnation for those who are in Christ Jesus. For the law of the Spirit of life in Christ Jesus has set you free from the law of sin and of death.
>   ROMANS 7:18–25; 8:1, 2 NAS

The Law

Frustration and depression result in religious groups' trying to live by an outward law. God's salvation is not dependent upon our keeping the outward law. This is not to say that Christians disregard the law of God, but rather that people do not become Christians or remain Christians by their own power and religiosity.

The passage cited from Romans records the frustration that resulted in the Apostle Paul when he tried to keep the law in his own power. The Christian life is a supernatural life and can only be lived by the power of Christ. An individual trying to please God by his own efforts "cannot please God" (*see* Romans 8:8 NAS).

The Spirit World

Much counsel has been directed at the soul of man. However, the *spirit* is the innermost part of man and is the most important part in a Christian's search for freedom from frustration. Some people have turned to other spirits (evil spirits) for freedom from frustration. The rise of the occult is a mark of this generation. Feature articles have appeared in prominent magazines. The freedom obtained from other spirits is short-lived and results in destruction. I have had the experience of listening to young people who were at least to some degree involved in witchcraft. These young people shared a frightening story with frustrating results. Satan knows the importance of not only dealing with a person's soul (mind, will, and emotions) but also with his *spirit*.

If Christian counselors are to be effective, they must not only help their clients find psychological freedom, but they must realize that only Jesus can give and maintain real freedom and peace of mind. This peace of mind begins with a rebirth in one's spirit by accepting Christ and continues as Christ's influence spreads outward from the spirit to change the soul (mind, emotion, and will).

Part II

Recognizing Emotional Problems

For God hath not given us the spirit
of fear; but of power, and of love,
and a sound mind.

2 TIMOTHY 1:7

4 An Approach to Conceptualizing and Understanding Mental Illness

Definitions

The terms "mental health" and "mental illness" are used often
but are quite vague and general terms. These terms mean different things to different people. In fact, to a degree, they mean
different things to different psychiatrists. Thomas Detre and
Henry Jarecki give one of the best in-depth criteria we have read
concerning "mental health."[1] However, in brief, below are some
broad definitions and some areas of agreement among psychiatrists for diagnosing emotional problems.

An individual is considered mentally healthy if he is in contact
with reality and is sufficiently free of anxiety so that he is not
significantly incapacitated functionally, socially, or biologically
for any extended period of time. He is not so uncomfortable that
he develops a prolonged sleep problem, becomes socially withdrawn, and/or has trouble at his job. This individual can still
function emotionally without being unduly uncomfortable for a
prolonged period of time.

In contrast, an individual with a clear-cut mental health problem may have lost contact with reality; or be so filled with anxiety that he suffers significantly biologically, socially, and
functionally. Symptoms that all people have (anxiety, fear, depression, worry, guilt, body aches and pains, etc.) increase in

63

magnitude and occur more often in these individuals. Their biologic functions (sleep, appetite, sex) are impaired. Their social
interaction suffers. Other people may note that something seems
wrong. They may be functioning poorly in their jobs. If a person
has significant trouble in three basic areas (biologic, social, functional) beyond a transient period, he has a mental problem.
Below are a sample of the chief complaints of individuals who
did suffer significantly in these three areas:

"I feel unwanted."

"Not able to sleep . . . mind won't shut off at night."

"I stay depressed most of the time. I am very high-strung."

"Lonely and in pain."

"Recurring nightmares and listlessness. . . . I don't have any
real ambition."

"An inability to cope with stress."

"Fear of doing something . . . unreal feelings . . . wicked
dreams and thinking."

"Depression, apathy, loss of contact with reality."

"Life in general is dull or else threatening."

"Nervous."

"I feel symptoms of weakness and tiredness."

"Nervous tension and confusion."

"Depression and inner conflicts."

"Psychological addiction to intravenous amphetamines."

"Depression and drinking."

"I have what is called a dual personality."

"Dizziness, fainting spells."

"Headaches . . . unable to handle my father . . . he puts pressure on me about my marriage."

"Drinking since mother's death."

"Drinking to make my painful feelings go away."

Diagnosing Mental Problems

There are those who feel that psychological problems do not
exist. We believe this is due to a lack of understanding.

The mind, emotion, and will do exist, and problems in these
areas are what are referred to as psychological problems. By

biblical context, the soul is the mind, emotion, and will; and by biblical documentation even godly men had significant problems in one of these three areas resulting in depression (*see* Psalm 32) and even psychosis (*see* Daniel 5:21).

There are also those who suggest that psychiatric diagnoses should no longer be used but rather that degrees of irresponsibility should be determined. This would make communication among mental health workers such as psychiatrists, pastors, and social workers extremely difficult. Two terms such as *paranoid schizophrenia* or Alzheimer's dementia can tell us literally volumes, whereas a colleague stating that a patient was moderately irresponsible would indicate little clinically.

I agree that mental health workers should be extremely careful when using psychiatric diagnoses, but to go to the other extreme is equally harmful and unreasonable.

For organizational purposes, mental problems can be broken down into two broad categories: mental retardation and mental illness.

Mental Retardation

A person is considered mentally retarded if his I.Q. is 85 or below. The degree of retardation is designated as follows:

Type	I.Q.
Borderline mental retardation	68–85
Mild mental retardation	52–67
Moderate mental retardation	36–51
Severe mental retardation	20–35
Profound mental retardation	under 20

The causes of mental retardation are numerous: infection, intoxication, trauma, physical agent, disorder of metabolism, disorder of nutrition, brain disease, chromosomal abnormality, prematurity, and, psychosocial deprivation, among others.

Dr. Minirth relates the following case study to illustrate how mental retardation can overlap with other problems in a counselee.

CASE STUDY: Jeff was a fourteen-year-old boy brought in to see me by his father. The boy had a long history of both physical and emotional problems. Thus, the father desired a psychiatric evaluation. The father stated the boy first developed problems in the second grade after being hit by a car. This resulted in a blow to his head. Soon afterwards, the boy developed problems in school. Then he developed severe peptic ulcer disease and had had several surgeries for this. The evaluation revealed the boy had borderline mental retardation. He also had some schizophrenic symptoms. With supportive psychotherapy, antipsychotic medication, and appropriate school placement, he adjusted well. It was interesting to note in this case that one uncle also suffered from latent schizophrenia. Another interesting fact was the conflict that had existed between the patient and his parents. He had been smothered by one and deserted by the other.

Mental Illness

In conceptualizing mental illness and understanding how it develops along a continuum, we would offer Figure 1 as an overall format for understanding how life's pressures can develop into psychological stress. Stress can then precipitate significant anxiety, and this anxiety may subsequently be displaced into a wide variety of mental disorders.

When an individual feels overwhelmed by life's pressures, the cause may come from a variety of factors. Listed below are eight categories of "Life Pressures" that can serve to place the individual under substantial stress.

Life Pressures

1. Unpredictable events. It was noted years ago that major events that bring change into our lives exert a toll of stress. These events need not necessarily be negative to exert stress upon an individual; even very positive events such as getting married, being pregnant, or taking a vacation can serve to add up the points of stress in one's life. In 1967, Holmes and Rahe developed a stress rating scale that has become a benchmark standard in the field of psychology for ranking the impact of stressors in a counselee's recent life. The counselee is asked to

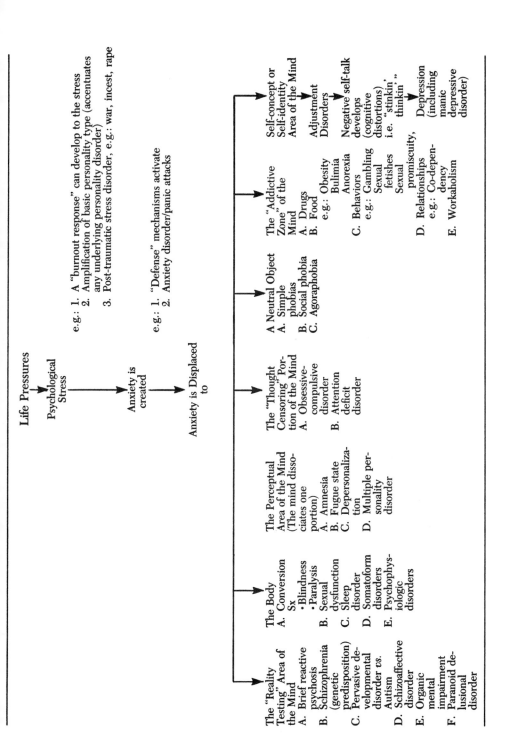

Life Pressures
↓
Psychological Stress

Anxiety is created → Anxiety is Displaced to

e.g.: 1. A "burnout response" can develop to the stress
2. Amplification of basic personality type (accentuates any underlying personality disorder)
3. Post-traumatic stress disorder, e.g.: war, incest, rape

e.g.: 1. "Defense" mechanisms activate
2. Anxiety disorder/panic attacks

The "Reality Testing" Area of the Mind
A. Brief reactive psychosis
B. Schizophrenia (genetic predisposition)
C. Pervasive developmental disorder vs. Autism
D. Schizoaffective disorder
E. Organic mental impairment
F. Paranoid delusional disorder

The Body
A. Conversion Sx
 • Blindness
 • Paralysis
B. Sexual dysfunction
C. Sleep disorder
D. Somatoform disorders
E. Psychophysiologic disorders

The Perceptual Area of the Mind (The mind dissociates one portion)
A. Amnesia
B. Fugue state
C. Depersonalization
D. Multiple personality disorder

The "Thought Censoring" Portion of the Mind
A. Obsessivecompulsive disorder
B. Attention deficit disorder

A Neutral Object
A. Simple phobias
B. Social phobia
C. Agoraphobia

The "Addictive Zone" of the Mind
A. Drugs
B. Food
 e.g.: Obesity
  Bulimia
  Anorexia
C. Behaviors
 e.g.: Gambling
  Sexual fetishes
  Sexual promiscuity,
D. Relationships
 e.g.: Co-dependency
E. Workaholism

Self-concept or Self-identity Area of the Mind
Adjustment Disorders
Negative self-talk develops (cognitive distortions) i.e. "stinkin' thinkin'"
Depression (including manic depressive disorder)

Figure 1

67

circle the events that have occurred in his or her life in the last twelve months. Then the corresponding values for these various events are added up and the totals are assessed in the following ways: If the score is 150 or less, there is less than a 30 percent chance of serious change in one's health in the next year. If the score is 150 to 300, then there is a 50 percent chance of serious change in one's health in the next year. If the score is 300 or greater, there is an 80 percent chance of a serious change in one's health in the next year.

Figure 2

HOLMES–RAHE SOCIAL READJUSTMENT
RATING SCALE

Test done in 1967. Ratings relate only to stresses undergone in the last twelve months.

EVENT	VALUE	SCORE
Death of spouse	100	
Divorce	73	
Marital separation	65	
Jail term	63	
Death of a close family member	63	
Personal injury or illness	53	
Marriage	50	
Fired at work	47	
Marital reconciliation	45	
Retirement	45	
Change of health of family member	44	
Pregnancy	40	
Sex difficulties	39	
Gain of a new family member	39	
Business adjustment	39	
Change in financial state	38	
Death of a close friend	37	
Change in line of work	36	
Change in number of arguments with spouse	35	
Mortgage over one-year's net salary	31	
Foreclosure on mortgage or loan	30	
Son or daughter leaving home	29	
Trouble with in-laws	29	
Outstanding personal achievement	29	
Spouse begins or stops work	26	

EVENT	VALUE	SCORE
Begin or end school	26	
Change in living conditions	25	
Revision of personal habits	24	
Trouble with boss	23	
Change in work hours or conditions	20	
Change in residence	20	
Change in schools	20	
Change in recreation	19	
Change in church activities	19	
Change in social activities	19	
Mortgage or loan less than one-year's net salary	17	
Change in sleeping habits	16	
Change in number of family get-togethers	15	
Change in eating habits	15	
Vacation	13	
Christmas	12	
Minor violations of the law	11	
Miscellaneous:	——	
	——	
	——	

Score total:
1. If you have 150 or less, there is a 30 percent chance of serious change in your health in the next year.
2. If you have a 150–300 score, there is a 50 percent chance of serious change in your health in the next year.
3. If you have a 300 score or greater, there is an 80 percent chance of a serious change in your health in the next year.

2. Unreasonable People. Dealing with unreasonable and overbearing individuals over a period of time can place a significant load of stress on a person, especially when these individuals have a large measure of effect on the person.

3. Unwise Priorities or Behaviors. This can involve the failure to use good decision-making skills, failure to appropriately arrange one's schedule to be consistent with chosen priorities, or even the effects of chronic communication problems.

4. Unscriptural Goals. Living outside of God's will when it comes to one's chosen goals and objectives for life can lead to significant stress.

5. Undealt-with Personal Issues. Items such as chronic anger, bitterness, or painful secrets that wear away at the inner soul of an individual can produce significant stress over a lengthy period.

6. An "Unrelenting" Temperament. Individuals who are particularly stress-prone and hard-driving are sometimes referred to in medical literature as Type A personalities. Such individuals are unrelenting and pressure-driven, and such temperament traits tend to put a tremendous amount of stress on the individual. They are often unrealistically ambitious and pursue goals in an inflexible fashion. They may show a sense of guilt when on vacation or taking time to personally relax. To others they sometimes appear to have an unrelenting need for power or recognition. They are tense physically and sometimes show such motions or gestures as facial grimacing, grinding of teeth, or TMJ syndrome. They may pound their fist, tap their feet, or play with a pencil in a rhythmic fashion. They are frequently impatient and push for speed. Their conversation is frequently characterized by bursts of rapid speech, varying in volume and pitch; and they frequently are poor listeners. They come across as self-centered and are prone to push others as hard as they push themselves. They may react impulsively or quickly when unpredicted events occur, and they seem to be able to simultaneously follow several lines of reasoning or trains of thought at once. They pride themselves in persistence and being able to anticipate circumstances before they occur; and yet they live with the constant dread that they are not taking appropriate notice of the unseen signs of some impending calamity coming their way.

These individuals with an unrelenting temperament tend to emotionally react before they have thought situations through. The following four steps have proven helpful in reducing stress in these individuals by assisting them to understand in any situation: (1) what happened, (2) how I felt, (3) what I did, and (4) the result. Marilee Horton, a friend and lay counselor, who has helped many women individually and in her seminars, feels that these steps have been a very effective tool for her over the years.

7. Unhealthy Management of Our Physical Body. Medical science has known for many years that the proper maintenance of fitness, exercise, rest, and nutrition all play a major role in reducing the deleterious effects of stress on the fabric of the human personality. There is even evidence now that our immune system and our capacity to resist certain types of cancer may be positively affected by correct exercise, nutrition, and the reduction of stress in our lives.

8. Unwillingness to Yield to God. There is probably nothing more stressful in an individual's life than to have an issue of nonresolution between oneself and God. When God has an agenda to deal with a certain element in our lives or change a certain behavior, to resist His will can bring persistent and insurmountable stress into our lives. Some counselees have been holding back on God in an area of their personality for years and only when this "holdout" is ceased will they be able to experience a measurable reduction in stress in their life.

Psychological Stress

When these life pressures mount to a point of significant intensity from any combination of the eight areas mentioned above, a state of chronic and often profound psychological stress may result. Such psychological stress can cause any number of problems for the counselee, but at least three major outcomes may occur.

Outcome Number 1

The most common outcome of chronic psychological stress is a gradual "burnout response" to this stress. This emotional burnout can occur in any individual who is exposed to significant psychological stress over an extended period of time. Hans Selye describes a sequence of stages that the body passes through

when responding to a particularly intense level of stress. First is
the alarm reaction, followed by the stage of *resistance,* and then
eventually the stage of *exhaustion* follows. In this last stage of
exhaustion, the individual is vulnerable to forces that would
serve to wear him down psychologically, spiritually, or physically, and the individual is unable to respond to additional
stressors.[2]

The following twelve items are frequently seen as symptoms
of the burnout response to stress.

1. Exhaustion (A sense of tiredness, trouble keeping up with
   usual activities)
2. Detachment (Putting distance between self and others, less
   time and energy for relationships)
3. Cynicism (Boredom and/or disillusionment, questioning the
   value of God, friendships, activities)
4. Irritability and Impatience (There is a decrease in one's
   ability to accomplish objectives and individual may "turn on
   others.")
5. Sense of omnipotence ("Only I can do it right, nobody else
   can.")
6. Feeling unappreciated (More and more resentment about
   demands made, but the individual can't seem to say no.)
7. Subtle irresponsibility (Problem-oriented approach to tasks,
   negativism)
8. Paranoia (Feeling others are beginning to consistently work
   against you)
9. Decreased concentration and increased difficulty making
   decisions (Feeling indecisive and fearing that one will "fal-
   ter under pressure")
10. Psychosomatic afflictions and illnesses (Real illnesses
    brought on or worsened by psychological stress, such as
    chronic headaches, arthritis, diabetes, allergies, lingering
    colds, increased blood pressure, etc.)
11. Acting out (Expressing frustration and burnout through al-
    cohol consumption, promiscuity, spending sprees, gam-
    bling, etc.)

12. Bitterness (Chronic unforgiveness of others or the conditional acceptance of others, commonly associated with perpetual jealousy or envy)

Outcome Number 2

If there are tendencies toward a personality dysfunction or disorder, then these tendencies may be amplified. When this occurs, a person may evidence enough of the characteristics of the personality dysfunction to warrant having a diagnosis of personality disorder. A variety of personality disorders are recognized by the American Psychiatric Association as reflected in the *Diagnostic and Statistical Manual*, Third Edition, Revised (DSM III-R). Below are nineteen different types of personality disorders that can be accentuated or increased in expression when a person is undergoing significant psychological stress.

1. Paranoid Personality Disorder. Personality disorders characterized by a pervasive and unwarranted tendency to interpret the actions of other people as intentionally threatening. This usually begins in early adulthood and can be present in a variety of contexts. These individuals do not normally seek clinical attention, they tend to avoid intimacy, and the disorder is more common in men. Paranoid patients frequently tend to "personalize" coincidental or calamitous events.

CASE STUDY: Ed felt the Mafia was after him. Although the man had no evidence for his fear and although the interviewer explained in a very logical manner to Ed why the Mafia could not be after him, Ed felt firmly that this was the case and held to his delusion. Other than this one delusional system, Ed related well and his associations were appropriate.

2. Schizoid Personality Disorder. This individual has a consistent pattern of relative indifference to relationships with others and has a restricted range of emotional expression. He is also frequently unable to feel emotionally close to others.

Individuals with this disorder frequently lack social skills, finding it difficult not only to express intimacy but also to appropriately express hostility or assertiveness. They find it quite difficult to socialize with others and are seen sometimes as "cold fish," being indifferent to the praise and criticism of others.

3. Schizotypal Personality Disorder. Individuals with this personality disorder are seen as particularly peculiar. They may have rather odd beliefs, some paranoid suspiciousness, and sometimes fantasy-oriented or bizarre thought processes. Individuals with this disorder frequently appear eccentric or strange in their behavior and appearance, and may be unkempt in their personal hygiene and display unusual mannerisms. Sometimes they are known to talk to themselves and to be quite superstitious or feel that they have special "powers" that distinguish them from other individuals. Under significant stress, they may become psychotic at times, their social function is normally impaired, and they tend to have difficulty in the workplace. They are not uncommonly related to individuals who have true schizophrenia.

4. Anti-social Personality Disorder. Individuals with this personality disorder tend to have a consistent pattern of irresponsibility. They may have frequent initiation of fights with others and running away from home. They have difficulty conforming to the norms of social conduct with respect to submitting to authority, and they are frequently irritable and aggressive. They may fail to carry out financial obligations, tend to not have a very high regard for the truth, and are a bit reckless in their concern for either their personal safety or the safety of others. They tend to lack remorse or guilt about trespasses, and they have difficulty sustaining consistent work behavior. They are frequently absent from work and employers may see them as devious or shiftless. They tend not to be able to maintain consistent relationships for lengthy periods of time. They frequently have trouble with the law, sometimes coming from homes where there was either a neglectful or cruel or intensely critical parental treatment. Dr. Minirth recounts one case of a young man as follows: "I recall one young man who was on his way to prison if he should do anything else in conflict with the law. The patient seemed to feel no guilt and did not learn from his experience. He continued to be irresponsible and do things in direct conflict with the authorities. He was eventually sent to prison." Individuals with this personality type tend to reflect many of the characteristics described in Romans 1, of the "reprobate mind." In Romans 1 the following terms are used to describe the reprobate mind: unrighteous, wicked, covetous, malicious, full of envy, murder, deceit, and without understanding (vv. 29–31).

5. Borderline Personality Disorder. The definition of borderline personality disorder has really been most fully developed in the last five to seven years as a clearer understanding of this debilitating dysfunction has become available. An individual with a borderline personality has traditionally undergone some rather severe experiences in the early childhood years in which he developed deep insecurities of the personality that function around the issues of trust and the reliability of others. Borderline individuals have frequently been abused either physically, emotionally, or sexually. Their moods show a lot of instability, and they have tremendous difficulty maintaining stable relationships with others. They tend to get very close to and almost emotionally "suffocate" certain individuals. They then become frightened at the first hint that the relationship may be cooling off and tend to push that other individual away in intense anger. They seek to avoid painful feelings by "numbness" and deep personalization, and they may even turn to self-injurious behavior such as wrist scratching in order to help numb emotional pain through the superimposing of physical pain. Treating the borderline personality can be a long and difficult undertaking, but good treatment programs can result in substantial improvement in the quality of life that these individuals experience.

6. Histrionic Personality Disorder. The histrionic personality has the persistent pattern of attention seeking and excessive emotionality. This often begins in the teenage years, as they seek or demand reassurance of approval from others, and are sometimes called "praiseaholics." They may shift moods rapidly and show a rather shallow expression of emotions. They tend to be self-centered and have little tolerance for delayed gratification and frustration. They are characteristically attractive, can be seductive, and tend toward the flamboyant. They may be overly concerned with their physical appearance. Others often see them as charming and superficially appealing but lacking true genuineness. They form quick friendships but not very deep ones. They may attempt to keep others interested in them by presenting themselves as helpless or dependent on other individuals. Their actions may show significant inconsistency with their professed values or beliefs. Flights into romantic fantasy are seen often, and in fact sometimes histrionic individuals are prone to promiscuity. They may be naive about the consequences of this behavior trait and the effects that their seductive actions have on others. The tendency to develop multiple complaints of poor health such as headaches, chronic fatigue, or weakness beset these individuals. They may interestingly show a phenomenon called "la belle indifference," in which they speak poignantly and dramatically about the painfulness or suffering they are undergoing because of some physical malady; although their words reflect duress, their facial expressions and overall demeanor show almost a casual air of indifference and contentment with the whole situation.

CASE STUDY: Pauline complained mostly of anxiety. She presented her story rather dramatically and was attention seeking and seductive in her actions. She gave a history of emotional instability and over-reactivity. She seemed immature and self-centered. The psychiatric history revealed several important facts. First, she had been married once but had been unfaithful to her husband numerous times. She had also attempted suicide several times. She noted that early in her childhood, attention had been given her only when she was seen as pretty or when she could attract the favor of young men through her flirtatious behavior.

7. Narcissistic Personality Disorder. This personality disorder reflects individuals who are very sensitive to the criticism of others and see themselves consistently in a grandiose position of self-importance. Frequently, this belies an underlying sense of unworthiness. They fantasize about having unlimited power, beauty, or brilliance and are frequently in relationships that are self-gratifying superficially but invariably disturbed with empathy lacking. Others see them as presumptive, exploiting relationships, carrying themselves with a sense of entitlement. Friendships are often entered into either consciously or unconsciously with the attitude, "What can I get out of this?" Others tend to think of narcissistic personality disorders as selfish, immature, and moody individuals who have to have things their way before they can get along with others. They tend to be confused and angry and blame others when they are rejected or avoided by someone because of their obnoxious behavior.

8. Avoidant Personality Disorder. The avoidant personality is characteristic of an individual who is seen as timid, has a significant fear of being rejected by others, and is uncomfortable in social situations. Such individuals generally avoid relationships unless they can feel very comfortable that they will be accepted in an uncritical fashion. They may not have any very close friends or confidence in relationships other than with relatives or individuals with whom they have had a long association. Those with avoidant personalities yearn for acceptance and relationships with others, which helps distinguish them from schizoid personality disorders, who are relatively content being socially isolated. Avoidant personalities tend to fear being embarrassed or blushing in front of others.

9. Dependent Personality Disorder. The dependent personality disorder is reflective of an individual who demonstrates a pervasive pattern of finding it difficult to make decisions without excessive amounts of advice and reassurance from other individuals. These people characteristically show a profile of submissive behavior to others. They are frequently hurt by disapproval and are sensitive to criticism, especially when they feel they have been too forward or assertive. They tend to agree with the statements of others, even when they feel those statements are wrong. This agreement seems to be a desire to not be rejected. They sometimes feel helpless or vulnerable when they are alone, and they are easily discouraged and hurt deeply when relationships end, as this provokes their fear of being abandoned.

10. Obsessive-Compulsive Personality Disorder. The obsessive-compulsive personality is very common in Western culture, especially in the portions of society where there is a strong emphasis on the "work ethic." These individuals tend to have encountered significant discipline during the developmental years. Their family life is characterized by the constraining of emotions and personally being "in full control of one's self at all times." They tend to strive for perfection and are frequently intellectual, concerned more with facts and not feelings. They have trouble expressing how they really feel but they are great at intellectualization. They may seem cold, formal, and rigid. They are very invested in being in control of knowing their emotions but are also frequently stingy, even miserly, and may be obsessed with cleanliness. They are often concerned that they have never done enough at their work and they certainly live with a performance-based self-acceptance. Extreme cases of obsessive-compulsive personality can progress to the point of being diagnosed as an obsessive-compulsive disorder, which will be discussed later in this chapter.

CASE STUDY: Sam was very successful in the business world. He was successful because of his perfectionism. However, his being perfectionistic had begun to get him into trouble. He could no longer relax. He was having trouble controlling his anger. Through therapy, he began to relax more and stopped carrying his perfectionism to the extent of being overly dutiful, overly conscientious, and overly concerned. It resolved many internal conflicts and thereby controlled his anger in a healthier fashion. He stopped worrying so much about what others thought.

11. Passive-Aggressive Personality Disorder. Individuals with the passive-aggressive personality express resistance and contempt for authority figures indirectly rather than directly. They fear direct aggression or assertiveness against perceived authority figures and, therefore, these indirect methods of sabotage or resistance may take the form of procrastination, stubbornness, "forgetfulness," and unexplainable inefficiency. They tend to pout, put things off, and be late. They are very prone to gossiping about others whom they perceive to be in authority or making demands upon them. They easily show resentment and are typically somewhat pessimistic about the future. They tend to present themselves as polite and easygoing, but this frequently is a facade for their underlying resentment. Dr. Minirth shares such an example.

CASE STUDY: I had been in therapy with Jack, a teenage boy, for several sessions. I had tried everything I knew to get the boy to open up, but he would not. He was determined to be passive-aggressive, as teenagers often are. I decided I would be passive also and not speak until he did. After ten minutes or so, my supervisor (during my residency) interrupted. We were making him nervous. This is often the case in therapy with passive-aggressive individuals. They can be hard to work with at times and may appear to delight in foiling the best attempts of others to help them.

12. PMS (premenstrual syndrome) Personality Disruption. This personality disruption is associated with females encountering the hormonal changes that occur roughly between the time of ovulation in midmenstrual cycle and the onset of menses itself. There are a wide variety of symptoms that can occur during this period of time. However, women who are experiencing PMS can clearly relate the cluster of debilitating emotional changes that surface. There is frequently a loss of energy, difficulty in concentrating, extreme irritability, impulsiveness, and a tendency to ruminate on self-critical fault patterns. Individuals may physically feel bloated, have headaches, and have joint or muscle pain and also be short-tempered and easily affected emotionally by others. Extreme mood swings from tearfulness to anger to sullen withdrawal and a sense of guilt and embarrassment are common. The hallmark of the PMS personality changes is that they are consistently linked to a specific time frame during the menstrual cycle and remit within a few days after the onset of the menstrual flow.

Another requirement for the diagnosis of a PMS personality disruption is that there are no other major psychiatric factors to account for these mood changes such as panic disorder, major depressive disorder, manic depressive disorder, or multiple-personality syndrome.

13. Sadistic Personality Syndrome. The sadistic personality syndrome is essentially a personality disorder characterized by aggressiveness and cruelty to others. These individuals may selectively show their aggressiveness and their cruelty to certain individuals while not being violent or aggressive with certain other individuals. They tend to be fascinated by violence, martial arts, or torture. They may resort to intimidation to get their way and may be amused at the suffering of others or cruelty to animals. These individuals rarely display their true nature when relating to individuals in positions of authority but tend to be more sadistic and cruel to family members or those who are their subordinates.

14. Self-Defeating Personality Disorder. The self-defeating personality disorder is reflective of individuals who tend to be drawn into relationships in which they are victimized. They will actually appear to be preventing others from helping them and are masters at replying to offers of suggested solutions to problems with "yes, but . . ." answers. They tend to exclude themselves from pleasurable activities and actually feel relieved when they are struggling and experiencing painful consequences. As mentioned above, they tend to avoid opportunities for pleasurable activities and act in such a way as to frequently cause others to reject them or to be angry with them. They tend to involve themselves in activities where they help others at the expense of pervasive self-sacrifice, even when such sacrifices are neither requested nor necessary under the circumstances. It can be stated that these individuals "snatch defeat from the jaws of victory."

15. Organic Personality Disorder. The organic personality syndrome is a persistent disturbance of personality that is due to some specific physical, that is, organic factor. Symptoms include recurrent outbursts of anger or aggressiveness, decreased evidences of social judgment, suspiciousness of others, and indifference. With injury to the frontal lobes, there typically is apathy and indifference, and an individual may lose interest in formerly pleasurable activities such as hobbies or socializing with others. Frequently they show difficulties with social judgment. They may behave in a belligerent way and tend to be intrusive and irritating to others. They may force their way into conversations or when engaging in interactions with others make inappropriate or rude remarks. They tend to exaggerate, be verbose, and be sensitive to criticism and even somewhat paranoid in their skepticism of the intentions of others. Individuals with organic personality syndrome, unlike individuals with general dementia, tend to have little impairment of memory and their abstract thinking may be relatively preserved. They frequently make mistakes socially in relationships with others and may be indiscreet in their behavior, such as making sexually provocative remarks at inappropriate times. As mentioned above, they can show aggression and anger that are significantly out of proportion to the precipitating events.

16. Multiple-Personality Disorder. The multiple-personality disorder is an unusual and striking disorder that appears to occur largely as a result of severe early-life psychological trauma, usually sexual and/or physical abuse. The pervading theory is that the vulnerable and still-developing personality of the child simply cannot handle the terrifying and overwhelming stress of the abusive situation in which the child is growing up; therefore, the child "splits" his or her world into various compartments so that some of these "compartments" are safe, while the fear and terror that is going on can be sealed off in other compartments. Typically these individuals have two or more distinct personalities and these personalities will emerge at different times to take control of the person's behavior. Not all multiple personalities are totally unaware of the existence of the different personalities. In fact, in the process of psychotherapy with multiple personality, there is usually a supervising personality that is generally aware of all the other personalities. The individual can reach a point at which they are quite conscious of when they are transitioning into the various personality states. Lengthy and intense psychotherapy by a qualified professional is generally required to successfully treat a true multiple-personality disorder.

17. Gender-Identity Disorder. Individuals with a gender-identity disorder generally speaking are either confused or highly conflicted about their sexual gender. A young man who is persistently and intensely distressed about being a male, who has an aversion to male clothing and insists on wearing stereotypical feminine clothing, and who decries his male anatomic features would be an example of a gender-identity disorder. These pervasive identity disorders usually surface in childhood during the prepubescent years. Transsexualism is a sense of discomfort or inappropriateness connected with one's sexual identity in an individual who has reached puberty. Individuals with this disorder frequently complain of feeling uncomfortable wearing the clothes of their assigned sex, and they tend to engage in activities that are culturally associated with activities of the opposite sex. They find their genitals repulsive and in extreme cases would alter their genitalia to that of the opposite sex. These have been referred to as "sex-change operations." Some gender-identity confusion is common in adolescent males and females during the turbulent preteenage and early teenage years. However, males who develop a persistently homosexual life-style and females who develop a lesbian life-style are manifesting a self-identity that is inconsistent with their innate gender configuration. Theories abound as to the actual etiological factors in the development of the homosexual or lesbian. We believe that the roots of the disorders stem from early difficulties in identifying with the same-sex parental figure and a subsequent compounding effect caused by the need for nurturance being confused with eroticism. What can develop then is a sense of the need for affection and "nurturance" from a caregiver being confused with the erotic need to somehow be sexually intimate with that individual. During the early and midteenage years, this attraction and confusion in self-identity can proceed to full-fledged homosexual experimentation and the development of virtually an addiction to either homosexual or lesbian activities. Homosexuality and lesbianism are difficult to treat and are deleterious addictions worthy of the most accomplished psychological and spiritual treatment available. The Scriptures certainly teach that the ongoing practice of homosexual or lesbian conduct is in contradiction to the basic tenets of biblical Christianity.

18. Cyclothymic Personality. These individuals are characterized by being either depressed, elated, or alternating between the two. When they are feeling high, these individuals have a bubbly personality and are outgoing and likable. They have a tremendous amount of energy and can be very successful. They are doing a dozen things at once. When these individuals are feeling low, they are sad, blue, and feel hopeless and helpless.

19. Explosive Personality. These individuals are emotionally explosive when provoked. They have outbursts of temper and may become violent. The individuals with these tendencies are frequently likable and have good personalities until put under emotional pressure.

Outcome Number 3

A third major outcome that can develop when an individual is under significant psychological stress is the development of a specific disorder known as a *post-traumatic stress disorder*. Post-traumatic stress disorder (PTSD) is a disorder that is brought on by an individual's experiencing an event that is outside the normal range of human experience. Such an event would be significantly distressing to almost anyone. Such events as the loss of a close loved one, sudden destruction of one's community, the experience of physical violence such as wartime carnage or being seriously assaulted would all qualify as events that could bring on a PTSD. The disorder is characterized by the event being regularly reexperienced in a variety of ways such as possible repetitive painful dreams of the event, intrusive and disruptive recollections of the event, or a sudden sensation as if the event

were somehow recurring. These recurrences are sometimes referred to as "flashbacks" to the episode and can be very intense.
Sometimes exposure to events that resemble or symbolize the
original trauma can provoke significant emotional distress. Also
these individuals will regularly tend to avoid activities or situations that arouse remembrance of the event. They may feel
detached from others, show a constricted range of emotional
expression, and report feeling "numb" emotionally. These individuals frequently muster efforts to avoid thoughts or feelings
related to the previous trauma, and they may have a sense of
negativism about their own future. Another symptom that is
seen with PTSD is persistently increased symptoms of arousal
such as an exaggerated startle response, irritability, difficulty
with sleep, and disruptive concentration. These individuals are
sometimes hypervigilant and may become very anxious with
dizziness, nausea, abdominal distress, chills, "lump in the
throat," and rapid heart rate when being exposed to events that
bring recollection of the previous traumatic incident. The general public's awareness of PTSD has been heightened significantly by the high visibility that the disorder has attained in
conjunction with its treatment in the Vietnam War veterans
returning to this country after combat.

When Anxiety Is Created at a Clinically Significant Level

Anxiety can be defined as "a diffuse, unpleasant uneasiness,
apprehension, or fearfulness stemming from anticipated danger,
the source of which is uncertain or unidentifiable."[3] In an effort
to decrease the intense level of anxiety now beginning to "leak"
through the interconscience level of dysfunction in the personality, the personality (usually unconsciously) begins to implement a series of "defensive mechanisms" designed to defend
against this anxiety by somehow changing the situation (or the
person's perception of the situation) so as to decrease its perceived level of threat or danger. An explanation of ten common
defense mechanisms that individual personalities implement in
emotional "self-defense" against anxiety follows.

Defense Mechanisms—Healthy and Unhealthy Ways to Handle Anxiety

The disorders we have described are typical chief complaints indicating anxiety. These anxieties were manifested in various problem types such as patients with depression, psychosis, and hysterical trends. In fact, the way anxiety is handled often determines the type of mental problem that develops. The particular way the individual handles the anxiety is determined by defense mechanisms.

Defense mechanisms often operate on a subconscious level. Thus, one may not be immediately aware of the reason he does something. And, if he is not careful, he may justify inappropriate behavior and even sin.

Some defense mechanisms are good and healthy, but others are not. For example, *projection* can be an unhealthy defense mechanism by which one attributes his own thoughts and feelings to someone else. A Christian who reacts drastically to specific faults in others may actually be projecting his own faults. In 1 Samuel 19 the story of Saul's wanting to kill David is recorded. Undoubtedly Saul felt very threatened by David and felt David wanted to do away with him. The truth was that Saul wanted to do away with David.

CASE STUDY: Jane stated that men *always* flirted with her. It may be that she was projecting her own desire to flirt and imagined the flirting was coming from the men.

In the above case, as in all cases presented, specific names and details are not used. In many, insignificant details have been changed or deleted.

A second defense mechanism is *reaction formation*. Through a reaction formation, an individual does exactly the opposite of what he would like to do. For example, a reformed alcoholic may become the spokesman in the community against alcohol. Also, a minister may evidence this if he repeatedly speaks against pornography. Some reaction formation is probably common to all our personalities, but the excessive and unknowing use of reaction formation to deal with emotional conflicts can be very detrimental. For example, in his effort to control his basic disdain for others, a sociopath might appear very religious. Clearly, the Pharisees were outwardly very pious, but inwardly they were struggling with drives and motives that were nearly reprobate. Another example is found in Proverbs 13:24 where the case of a parent who never spanks or disciplines his child is recorded. Hatred is said to be the reason for the lack of discipline. In other words, a parent who would literally like to beat his child to death may go to the opposite extreme and not spank at all.

CASE STUDY: Suzie was an eight-year-old girl who was repeatedly setting fire to the house. The mother refused to discipline the girl. Psychiatric evaluation and history revealed she had resentment toward the girl and was undergoing a reaction formation.

Rationalization is a defense mechanism that many use to avoid responsibility. Not only is there a danger of rationalizing irresponsibility but also sin. Abraham lied about his wife Sarah, David committed adultery with Bathsheba, and Solomon built temples for idols. Even these godly men rationalized to permit their behavior; yet, their rationalizations cost them much. Hopefully, we will learn from these lessons of history.

A fourth defense mechanism is *introjection*. Introjection is often used by depressed individuals to assume responsibility for events outside their realistic control. This explains why depressed individuals so often feel guilty when they are truly guiltless. Introjection in adults is usually unhealthy; however, one case when healthy introjection did occur in an adult was Christ's introjecting the responsibility for our sins upon himself (*see* Matthew 27:46).

CASE STUDY: Joe felt guilty when he found his boss having an affair. While having nothing to do with the whole situation, he felt personally responsible and guilty. "Maybe I could have done something to prevent it . . ." yet Joe never really had an opportunity to know about or to influence the situation.

A fifth defense mechanism that certainly should be mentioned is *repression*. Repression is basic to all other defense mechanisms. Repression is the involuntary exclusion of unwanted thoughts from consciousness. Thus, an unwanted thought, such as the true reason for an inappropriate behavior, is first repressed and then a second defense mechanism is used such as rationalization to justify the inappropriate behavior.

A sixth defense mechanism is *suppression*. Suppression is the conscious analogue of repression. It is the voluntary exclusion of unwanted thoughts from consciousness. To pay attention to one idea one must exclude many others that would pop into the mind. Students use suppression during Christmas holidays to enjoy the season and not worry about school. Of course, this is a healthy use of suppression.

A seventh defense mechanism is *compensation*. By compensation one excels in one area because he feels inferior in another.

CASE STUDY: Bill felt inadequate in sports. He compensated by making excellent grades in school.

An eighth defense mechanism is *idealization and identification*. This is the overestimation of desirable traits in another. Many students do this with their professors. Christians are particularly prone to find someone other than Christ to idealize. This is not to say that we should not identify with or imitate other Christians. Apostle Paul told the Philippians to imitate him as he imitated Christ (*see* Philippians 3:17).

Isolation is the splitting off of an emotion from an event or thought. By this, many individuals with obsessive-compulsive personalities avoid being in touch with their emotions. They seem to endure disturbing events with little emotions. Of course, the emotions are there; they are just not in touch with them.

Displacement defends the individual by shifting the emotional component of one event to another event or person. This explains why, when a man has a difficult day at work, he explodes at his wife the same night. Hysterics often displace anxiety onto their bodies by developing various physical problems.

Often, how and when they are applied determines whether they are healthy or unhealthy. Learning to sublimate our instinctive drives into actions for Christ is a step toward maturity. For example, the defense mechanism of *identification* may be healthy and is scriptural. The Apostle Paul asked others to imitate him as he imitated Christ.

Knowing the above and other basic defense mechanisms will help in considering the mental problems soon to be discussed. One can predict with a good deal of accuracy the defense mechanisms that will be used by an individual with a particular mental problem. For example, the hysteric will usually use denial and displacement. The obsessive-compulsive will usually use isolation, reaction formation, undoing, and magical thinking. The schizophrenic uses fantasy and regression. The paranoid uses projection. The depressed person uses introjection frequently.

Anxiety Disorders

When significant levels of anxiety begin to accumulate in a person's personality despite the personality's defense mechanism trying to attenuate this anxiety, then various types of "anxiety disorders" can break through and begin to occur. Two of the most common of these anxiety disorders are generalized anxiety disorder and panic attacks. The generalized anxiety disorder is characterized by extensive worry and large amounts of fearfulness about several life circumstances, for example, worrying about finances when finances are in no distinct jeopardy and unfounded concerns about the welfare of one's loved ones where there is no actual threat to their well-being. To qualify as a generalized anxiety disorder, these symptoms should be in occurrence for a period of at least six months. There are general problems with many of the following symptoms including increased muscle tension with frequent restlessness and ease in fatigue. The individual frequently reports "feeling shaky." There is a sense of being "keyed up," feeling on edge, and frequently problems with concentration and disrupted attention span due to anxiety. The individual may have trouble falling asleep or staying asleep, and there is increased irritability and decreased frustration tolerance. The individual may complain of dizziness or light-headedness. There is frequently some abdominal distress such as chronic heartburn, nausea, or diarrhea. There may be stomach cramps, dry mouth, sweaty palms, heart palpitations, and shortness of breath along with frequent urination and a "lump in the throat." These individuals report feeling tense, restless, and nervous to the point of being near the limits of their tolerance.

Panic attacks bear some obvious similarity to the generalized anxiety disorder, but there are distinguishing features. These panic attacks are distinct periods of intense discomfort and fearfulness. They are unexpected and not brought on by the exposure to a specifically strong event that would normally cause anxiety. To qualify as a panic attack, several of the following symptoms should be occurring: trembling or shakiness, sweating, a sense of choking, shortness of breath frequently with a sensation of smothering, some chest pain or discomfort with heart palpitations or rapid heart rate, a sense of fear of dying or "losing one's mind," and frequently numbness and tingling sensation in the hands, feet, or face. Sometimes individuals will also feel abdominal distress, nausea, or diarrhea and possibly experience hot flashes with chills and/or dizziness and faintness as well. Panic attack, as mentioned above, usually develops suddenly with several of the symptoms and will increase in intensity within approximately ten minutes of the beginning of the initial appearance of the symptoms. The episode cannot have been brought on by a clear-cut physical precipitant, such as hyperthyroidism or caffeinism. Occasionally a heart condition known as mitral valve prolapse can be associated with the development of panic disorders. Panic disorders may occur with or without agoraphobia being present, a disorder which will be discussed later in this chapter.

Disorders Occurring When Anxiety Becomes Displaced

As indicated in Figure 1 earlier m this chapter, when pressures and problems precipitate significant psychological stress

and that psychological stress creates anxiety that is not able to be
dispelled, then the anxiety may eventually be displaced into one
or more areas of mental functioning. Of course, these areas are
not anatomically discrete areas nor are they precisely distinctive
and exclusive of overlap. However, the conceptualization of
problems forming into psychological stress, then creating anxiety, and this anxiety eventually being displaced and contributing to the formation of a variety of mental disorders is a helpful
conceptual paradigm. The following seven groupings of mental
disorders are those groupings found in Figure 1 earlier in this
chapter.

I. The "Reality Testing" Area of the Mind

When anxiety is displaced to the so-called "reality testing
area" of the mind, psychotic features can develop. These psychotic reactions can range from the *brief reactive psychosis* that
appears to be almost totally the result of intense external anxiety
overwhelming a person's normal psychological coping mechanisms, to the *long-term schizophrenic disorders* that appear to
be highly influenced by genetically inherited predispositions to
develop such a disorder. Psychosis is essentially a loss of touch
with reality. It affects several areas of the individual's ability to
function, including the content of the individual's thought, frequently with multiple fragmented and bizarre thought patterns.
For example, an individual may have an implausible belief that
other individuals are reading his mind or that his thoughts are
being transmitted somehow through the television set. Individuals with bizarre thought content may feel controlled by external
forces or they may have delusional ideas about their own abilities, seeing themselves as developing a "messiah complex."
Their form of thought may be disruptive, too, wherein their
speech may be disorganized, rambling from subject to subject,
pressured to a pace that is not understandable or demonstrating
the use of bizarre words that do not convey the information
needed. They may have thought blockage in that they are able
to speak only a few words and then their thoughts and speech
come to an abrupt halt, usually followed by distractions to an-

other subject, then picking up with a new train of thought. Their perception of their environment may be distorted, primarily with hallucinations. Auditory hallucinations (hearing voices externally coming from nonexistent sources) is the most common form of hallucination, but there may also be visual hallucinations where the individual sees images, faces, or some other form of bizarre visual phenomena going on in his environment. Usually visual hallucinations indicate an organic injury to the brain, such as a drug reaction or post stroke confusion. There can also be hallucinations of smell, taste, and touch where an individual is totally convinced that strange and possibly poisonous odors are being vented into his home or workplace. Individuals withdrawing from various drugs, for example, may also feel that snakes or bugs are crawling on their bodies. If there are visual hallucinations, then they actually believe they see these animals tormenting them on their bodies. The person's emotional state is frequently affected, and he may have extreme mood swings with inappropriate laughter, loud speech, or aggressiveness alternating with sadness, withdrawal, and intense despondency. Sometimes with psychosis, especially with schizophrenia, there is a flattening of the affect where an individual seems almost robot-like in his emotional expression, although he may physically be quite active. The individual's sense of self is frequently disrupted in that he is not sure whether he is truly controlling events in his environment or they are controlling him. He may even feel that other individuals are somehow possessing or indwelling his body, which has been referred to as a "loss of ego boundaries." The individual may have difficulty initiating and maintaining goal-directed behavior and struggle with following through on a course of action that requires formal thought or personal reflection to thoughtfully gain the desired result. These individuals may be negativistic, refusing and resisting suggestions or directions from the outside, although they rarely have a viable alternative to the suggestions. They may well be preoccupied with illogical ideas, fantasies, and internal distortions that exclude appropriate communication and interaction with the outside world. Sometimes individuals with an acute psychosis may sit and rock back and forth or pace incessantly, talking to themselves and responding to auditory hallucinations as well as manifesting scattered and disorganized verbal productions. In cases of severe psychosis, personal hygiene (such as bathing habits or grooming habits) may deteriorate. Thus, individuals may appear disheveled in their dress and even foul smelling as their mental disorder makes it quite difficult for them to attend to their normal personal dress and hygiene needs as they ordinarily would.

With the brief reactive psychosis, the critical feature is that the psychotic symptoms begin after stress reaches an intense point, usually within several hours or up to one month after the onset of the intense stress or stressful event. Events are generally those that would cause intense stress to any normal person. There are frequently bizarre, even suicidal or aggressive, behavior and tremendous amounts of emotional disarray. The individual may require hospitalization or the use of antipsychotic medications. The favorable component of the disorder is that the individual usually will return to the baseline premorbid level of functioning after the brief reactive psychosis has passed.

The *schizophrenic disorders* are well-known psychiatric disorders that have been described for many years under a variety of different names. Schizophrenic disorders are described as being psychotic in their proportion and frequently manifested by disturbances that include perception, emotion and affect, behavioral patterns, communication, and language. These disruptions need to have been existent for at least six months. The thought disturbances frequently lead to the misinterpretation of reality, creating delusions as well. Commonly seen are loss of empathy for others, strong ambivalence about their own identity and selfhood, and auditory and visual hallucinations. Schizophrenia has a prevalence rate in the United States of between 0.6 and 3.0 percent of the population, thus affecting approximately 1.2 to 6 million Americans.[4] Schizophrenia can generally be broken down to five major categories as follows:

1. Paranoid Schizophrenia. This is characterized by the patient's being excessively suspicious and often hostile. The patient has the usual symptoms of schizophrenia, but he is also delusional and paranoid. He may really want to harm others, but he projects his feelings onto others and feels they want to harm him.

CASE STUDY: A middle-aged male came for an appointment because he was referred by a Christian Counseling Center. He presented the fear that his wife was trying to kill him. He had no proof of this, but his suspicions were strong. For example, his wife had asked for a vacation from her job. She had told him she wanted to take a vacation with him and get the marriage back together. When the wife commented that her boss had granted the vacation and even said, "Take however long it takes," the patient was sure the "it" meant she was going to kill him. He was also very worried about his wife's wedding vow, "Till death do us part." Subsequent psychiatric interviews revealed the extensive delusional system this patient had built. He also had a history of auditory hallucinations. He felt he had heard Christ speaking to him and calling his name. This patient had paranoid schizophrenia.

2. Undifferentiated Schizophrenia. Once referred to as simple schizophrenia, it can be characterized by social withdrawal, *regression*, and *autism*. Some hoboes or "street people" would fit this category.

CASE STUDY: A woman came for an appointment as an outpatient. She seemed shy, withdrawn, socially regressed, and autistic. She had never been able to hold a job for any length of time. She still lived with her parents, had very few, if any, close friends, and had never dated. Subsequent psychiatric evaluation revealed that this patient had simple schizophrenia. With supportive psychotherapy the patient did begin to improve.

Other individuals exhibiting a mix of schizophrenic symptoms that appear to be "stable" and fixed components of their personality may be described as chronic undifferentiated schizophrenics. These patients have various schizophrenic symptoms (paranoia, depression, withdrawal, etc.). Because of this variety of symptoms, they do not fit in any one particular category, so they are defined as an "undifferentiated type."

CASE STUDY: A patient had been in a psychiatric ward for twenty-five years. He was one of the few patients who had never been able to return home from the hospital. His loose associations, his inappropriate affect, and his bizarre behavior had gone on so long that they had been ingrained into his personality He was one of the sad cases who had suffered from chronic, undifferentiated schizophrenia.

3. Disorganized (or Hebephrenic) Schizophrenia. This is characterized by silliness and extreme regression.

CASE STUDY: A thirteen-year-old girl was brought by her parents for an evaluation. The parents said that the girl had always been a quiet girl, but very stable. She had suddenly started acting in a strange and irrational manner.

Upon psychiatric evaluation, she would not respond appropriately to questions. Her facial expression was extremely inappropriate. She would stand in front of a mirror and giggle as she gazed at herself.

The patient was found to have schizophrenia, childhood type because she was very young. However, she had hebephrenic symptoms

4. Catatonic Schizophrenia. This may be characterized by extreme withdrawal to the degree that the patient will not even move. By contrast, some catatonics may become very excited with much uncontrolled activity.

CASE STUDY: A young lady was admitted to a psychiatric ward because of her sudden break with reality. She was extremely withdrawn. In fact, she would maintain her extremities in whatever position they were placed.

On the other hand, another schizophrenic patient had to be watched carefully to keep him from harming himself by suddenly falling backwards or making some other excitatory movement.

The first case illustrates the *withdrawn* catatonic schizophrenic, while the second case illustrates the *excited* catatonic schizophrenic.

5. Residual Schizophrenia. This diagnosis is reserved for patients who have had psychotic breaks but are no longer overtly schizophrenic.

CASE STUDY: A twenty-eight-year-old black female came to my office with the desire to start psychotherapy. She gave a history of having had a psychotic break at one time. During that time, she heard voices, had a rich fantasy life, showed poor judgment, and did strange things like walk around the block in her pajamas. At the time of the interview, she was not overtly psychotic. However, her associations did seem a little loose, and her affect was a little inappropriate. Psychiatric evaluation revealed she had residual schizophrenia.

This patient's history was very interesting and deserves comment, for it shows the danger of an unstable early environment. Her mother and father divorced when she was very young. She moved often as she was growing up, first living with both her mother and father, then only with her mother, then with her grandparents, and then with her step-father. Her uncle tried to rape her when she was twelve years old. Her mother drank a lot. The history goes on and on in this fashion.

Of course, Christ did change the direction of her life. She became a Christian around twelve years of age and grew both spiritually and emotionally through her involvement in a local church.

Note: When there are major functional impairments in the mental operations of the preteenage child, such terms as childhood schizophrenia or childhood psychosis were previously utilized. These names have now been replaced by a more inclusive term, *Pervasive Developmental Disorder of Childhood.* The child with pervasive developmental disorder may show symptoms reminiscent of some or all of the symptoms of the adult schizophrenias. Also, he should be distinguished from the youngster with *Childhood Autistic Disorder.*

CASE STUDY: James was a ten-year-old white male who had been admitted to the psychiatric unit at the request of state authorities. James had threatened to kill his mother and grandmother with a shotgun. James had always related very poorly with his peers and was socially very regressed. Although he was socially very regressed, he did run the home and would become enraged when his desires were thwarted. Psychiatric evaluation revealed that he had extremely poor judgment, was very autistic, and was not in contact with reality.

The child with *Autistic Disorder,* however, would exhibit some of the following symptoms. He shows an impairment in his reciprocal social interaction that is the inability to successfully and with emotional empathy engage his environment. There is a lack of awareness of the feelings of others or even the existence of these feelings. He apparently has no concept of the need of others for privacy. There is frequently little or no imitation; for example, the child may not wave bye-bye or does not copy a mother's or father's normal household activities. There is little social play, and the child does not actively participate in simple games but prefers solitary endeavors. There is gross impairment in the ability to make friends with one's peer group, and the child demonstrates a lack of understanding of the norms and conventional guidelines in social interactions. The child frequently does not seek comfort at times of distress; for example, the child will not readily come to a parent when hurt, tired, or ill. The child may in fact repeat a stereotypic phrase when injured that does not directly relate to the injury, such as repeating "the TV, the TV, the TV" when seeking comfort for a stubbed toe. These children may stiffen when they are held and do not look for smiles or other social cues from adults making a social approach to the child. There is an absence of activities reflective of imagination such as play-acting adult roles or imitating fantasy characters. There are also abnormalities in the production of speech (rhythm and pitch of speech). The child may maintain a high pitch or monotonous tone of speech. These children show a distress over changes in rather trivial aspects of the environment and may become quite disorganized and disrupted by alterations to their routine. They have restricted range of interest and seem to be preoccupied with narrow interests. They may have some stereotyped body movements such as spinning or twisting and participation in head-banging. They appear to be preoccupied with repetitive sensory experiences such as feeling a textured material or being infatuated with the wheel on a play car, spinning it around over and over again.

Schizoaffective Disorder has been used to denote an individual who has a distinct mixture of schizophrenic symptoms as well as recurrent either manic or depressive symptoms. These individuals may alternate between being very euphoric and very depressed. A distinguishing mark with these patients is that, even when their mood swings are under control, they still exhibit various symptoms reflective of schizophrenia. On the other hand, when their schizophrenic symptoms are under control and they are not particularly bizarre or delusional, they may be plagued by ongoing mood swings that are still problematic. When medications are utilized with these individuals, they typically require a combination of medications that both assist in stabilizing their mood swings and serve to clarify their thought processes and reduce the cognitive distortions therein.

Psychosis can also be largely the function of *organic or physical mental impairments* that affect the brain. Anxiety that is overwhelming a person's defense mechanism may significantly worsen any underlying organic mental impairment. The five cardinal symptoms of organic brain syndrome or dementia are impaired intellect, impaired memory, a flattened or labile affect, impaired judgment, and disruptions in orientation. Individuals with organic brain syndrome or dementia may have either psychotic or nonpsychotic symptoms, and the condition may be either acute or chronic. The causes of the condition can be many, including alcohol, drugs, syphilis, encephalitis, or presenile dementia (for example, Pick's disease, Jakob-Creutzfeldt disease), senile dementia not otherwise specified, multi-infarct dementia, and primary dementia of the Alzheimer's type. Also epilepsy, metabolic disorders, and even toxic responses to environmental agents or medications can lead to organic brain changes. Patients with organisity characteristically tend to have difficulty repeating digits in reverse order after the counselor and struggle to remember four or five objects after a few minutes. They also have difficulty doing serial –7 subtractions (the patient is asked to begin with the number 100 and then subtract 7 from 100 and then 7 from the answer given and then 7 from the following answer, etc., until they go as far as they can). Patients with organic brain syndrome typically have difficulty going beyond the first two or three subtractions. An example of a psychotic organic brain syndrome or dementia is given in the case below.

CASE STUDY: A man concerned about his mother brought her to see us because he had noted her memory beginning to get progressively worse over the last two to three years. The patient was a widow living by herself but had been active with friends both in her community and in church. In the last several months, she had not only had worsening problems with her memory but had begun to isolate herself from her friends. Her son noticed she was not fixing meals anymore, and she was hoarding groceries and keeping perishable items such as milk and fresh vegetables and meat stacked in corners throughout the house. She then began to yell out at neighborhood children playing in the yard, accusing them of being sent to "spy on her." She would be up late at night phoning the police that "wild dogs" were trying to break into her home. She frequently wrapped herself in a blanket and walked through the house with a large stick, seeking the source of what she described as "demonic voices." She also had been seeing the faces of friends and enemies from her lifetime appearing on the walls of her home. She would go for days without changing clothes or bathing. She was unable on a clinical interview to orient herself to the time or place of the interview setting. She frequently spoke in phrases that were unrelated to the content of the interview situation and mumbled in response to auditory hallucinations. Her judgment and intellect were impaired, and she was not able to concentrate very well. She was frightened, anxious, and convinced that the doctors had been sent by her family to "steal her brain" so the family could have her inheritance, which was a pittance. The patient was subsequently diagnosed as having a psychotic organic brain syndrome (dementia) of the Alzheimer's type.

It is also known that specific injuries to the brain can cause mood disturbances. Research is still quite actively going on in this field to try to understand how specific brain impairments may lead to emotional or cognitive changes. For example, in a recent article in *The Psychiatric Times*, Robert Robinson, M.D., noted that "lesions of the left frontal cortex and left basal ganglia are the most likely injuries to produce major depressive disorder, while we have not found a strong association of minor depression with lesion location."[5]

Another psychotic disorder that can be aggravated by the personality being overloaded by intense anxiety is the *paranoid delusional disorder*. Paranoid delusional disorders are a form of psychosis. Obviously these patients have lost contact with reality through their paranoid delusions. While frequently having an elaborate delusional system, the patient typically has no other major mood or thought disorder. In other words, the paranoid ideation may be localized to a certain area of their lives and not appear to markedly affect their global functioning in other areas of their life-style.

II. The Body (Mental disorders that can arise when anxiety is displaced into the body)

One form of physical reaction to intense anxiety is the displacement of this anxiety into a particular body part or specific body function. The body then suffers a psychogenic loss of function. This loss of function may be blindness, deafness, paralysis, paresis, hemiplegia, aphasia, convulsions, or others. This is referred to in modern psychiatric terminology as a somatoform disorder of the *conversion type* (or hysterical neurosis, conversion type).

CASE STUDY: Miss L. was admitted to a psychiatric ward because of intense pain in her left leg. The pain was not related to any anatomical nerve distribution, and no significant organic pathology could be found on a physical examination or by X-ray. The young lady gave a life history of various body aches, pains, and symptoms. She was diagnosed with a hysterical neurosis, conversion type.

Another type of somatoform disorder is the *body dysmorphic disorder*. In this disorder, there is a preoccupation on the part of the patient with some defect that he imagines to be present in his appearance. It most commonly involves a flaw in facial appearance such as the shape of the nose, position of the ears, configuration of the jaw. This most commonly has its onset in his twenties or thirties.

A third type of somatoform disorder is *hypochondriasis* (known as hypochondriacal neurosis). These individuals have a persistent and very disconcerting fear that they are suffering from some serious disease, usually based on their own interpretation of various body sensations and perceived limitations of function. They may also have areas of pain that further lead them to believe that they have a disease that is persisting in spite of previous medical treatments. Attempts to reassure them by medical personnel usually are fruitless. These individuals are not delusional, and while they may be able to acknowledge that they could possibly be exaggerating the symptoms, they nevertheless are persistently concerned that there is some deep-seated physical problem.

The *somatization disorder* is similar to hypochondriasis and involves the individual's having multiple bodily complaints that have persisted for years, for which medical attention has been frequently sought, but for which there has not been a detectable physical cause noted. The individuals present the complaints in a vague or sometimes exaggerated way and are frequently cared for by a number of physicians. The individual will generally have complaints in multiple areas that may include abdominal pain, intermittent and difficult-to-identify problems, intolerance of foods from multiple food groups, amnesia, difficulty swallowing, double vision or blurred vision, burning sensation in the sexual organs or rectal area (other than during intercourse), painful menstruation, chest pain, joint and back pain, and also dizziness. Of course, these symptoms can relate to distinct medical problems, and a full medical workup must be implemented as a component of the overall workup of these patients.

The *somatoform pain disorder* is a disorder in which there is a preoccupation on the part of the patient with pain in the absence of definable physical causes for that pain. Appropriate medical evaluation will have uncovered no specific medical pathological process to account for the pain. On the other hand, if there is some medical cause noted for the pain, the usual finding is that the complaint of pain or the resulting work or social impairments from the pain are significantly in excess of the limitations that would normally be expected from the medical findings.

When anxiety is displaced into the body, a variety of otherwise normal body functions can be adversely affected. For example, there are a variety of *sexual dysfunctions*, including hypoactive sexual desire disorder, female sexual arousal disorder, male erectile disorder, inhibited female orgasm, inhibited male orgasm or premature ejaculation, and the sexual pain disorders such as dyspareunia and vaginismus. The specific treatment of severe sexual dysfunction is a fairly complex undertaking and may require specific professional intervention. Anxiety displaced into the body can result in a variety of *sleep disorders.* Some of these sleep disorders are related to congenital anatomic disruptions in the body's normal sleep-wake cycle, but superimposed anxiety can certainly aggravate and intensify an individual's sleep disorder. Such problems as primary insomnia, primary hypersomnia, sleep walking, sleep terrors, and nightmare disorder (dream anxiety disorder) are a few of the sleep disorders that are commonly encountered. The workup of a sleep disorder may require the patient's being evaluated in a sleep laboratory, which is available at most major medical centers, and can frequently arrive at a specific etiology for the individual's sleep dysfunction. Of course, when the sleep disorder is a result of anxiety arising from a known source or from depression, then treatment of the underlying psychological problem will frequently result in the correction of the sleep problem.

There are a variety of other miscellaneous somatoform disorders. In childhood, anxiety displaced into the body can sometimes contribute to the development of so-called *tic disorders.* These disorders may have an underlying genetic basis, however, which is known to worsen or exacerbate these tic disorders. The tic disorders include Tourette's syndrome, in which the tic (an involuntary recurrent, frequently rapid, and stereotyped motor movement or vocalization) will normally occur several times a day and the location, number, and frequency of the tic may change over time. To be classified as a tic, the behavior should not be associated with the use of any psychoactive substance nor any central nervous system disease such as encephalitis of a post-viral type or Huntington's chorea. In addition to Tourette's syndrome, there is also a transient tic disorder and a chronic motor or vocal tic disorder.

Anxiety displaced into the body can also present itself as an elimination disorder such as functional *encopresis,* in which the child passes feces into areas where it is not appropriate, for example, on the floor or in clothing. Very often the child feels quite ashamed or embarrassed by the encopresis and, as one might imagine, by humiliation at the hands of peers. Perceived inadequacy and damaged self-esteem is very common with this disorder. Functional *enuresis* is much more common than encopresis. The existence of any other complicating physical conditions (i.e., urinary tract infection, a seizure disorder, or diabetes) must be ruled out in making the diagnosis of functional enuresis. There appears to be some genetic pattern to this disorder since approximately 74 percent of all children with the disorder have a first-degree biological relative who has or has had the disorder.[6]

These disorders are also adversely affected by levels of anxiety that appear to quite negatively affect the child's capacity to speak properly. *Stuttering* is a speech disorder in which the individual experiences frequent repetitions or prolongations of sounds or syllables of words, and there is the resultant impairment in the fluency and flow of speech. Stuttering tends to affect males three times more frequently than females, and approximately 5 percent of children will stutter at some time in their development. It is more common in younger children, the prevalence in adults being approximately 1 percent.[7]

Cluttering is another form of speech disorder that can be adversely affected by anxiety and can certainly cause the child a tremendous amount of embarrassment and anxiety in and of itself due to adverse effects on the child's self-esteem. Cluttering usually begins after the age of seven and may make speech somewhat impaired in its intelligibility. Speech may be erratic and show disorganized rhythm, and there is frequently the presence of jerky spurts of speech that have somewhat inaccurate phrase patterns.

Elective mutism is the consistent refusal to talk in various social situations, generally including school. Yet the patient has the ability to comprehend both the written and spoken languages. It is found in fewer than 1 percent of children and is slightly more common in females than in males.

In addition to the above-mentioned adverse sequelae that can result from anxiety being displaced into the body, actual anatomical damage can be done to the body secondary to the effects of chronic stress and anxiety. With *psychophysiological disorders,* the autonomic nervous system, not the voluntary nervous system, is involved and stress is displaced in the autonomic nervous system. The autonomic nervous system is that part of the nervous system that regulates the vital functions of the body that are not controlled consciously, that is, those functions that are involuntary. The autonomic nervous system controls the activity of the smooth muscles of the digestive system, the glands of the body, and the activity of the heart itself. The autonomic nervous system controls both the sphincter muscles and narrow blood vessels and also raises blood pressure. The autonomic nervous system can also affect the level of tension within the deep muscles of the head, neck, and back. When the autonomic nervous system is involved, the patient could experience gastrointestinal dysfunction (ulcers, gastritis, constipation, colitis) or possibly respiratory disorder (asthma, hyperventilation, or hiccups, or even skin disorders such as pruritus and dermatitis).

Musculoskeletal disorders such as backaches or headaches can occur as well, including difficulties with arthritis. The sequence of problems arising from psychophysiological disorders can be diagramed as follows.

PSYCHOPHYSIOLOGIC DISORDERS

Hereditary Factors
↓
Early Environmental Factors (Social, Religious, Physical)
↓
Detrimental Defense Mechanism Develops at Early Age by Which
Anxiety Is Handled by Displacing It Onto a Body Function
↓
Acutely Stressful Situation
↓
Anxiety
↓
Hypothalamus of Brain Affected
↓
Autonomic Nervous System Affected
↓
Specific Organ Influenced
↓
Organ Pathology
↓
Psychophysiologic Disorder (Colitis, Ulcers, Asthma)

III. The Perceptual Area of the Mind

When significant amounts of anxiety are displaced in the perceptual area of the mind, the result can be *psychogenic amnesia*. This causes an individual to have a rather sudden inability to recall significant personal information from the past, which is too extensive to be explained by simple forgetfulness.

A psychogenic amnesiac may need to "block out" a particularly painful situation or set of circumstances. There are certain organic mental dysfunctions (such as substance abuse, intoxication from drugs, alcohol amnestic disorder, or even amnesia) that result from a concussion or epilepsy which must be ruled out. Psychogenic amnesia is rarely seen in the elderly, while most commonly observed in adolescent and young adult females. The amnesia usually follows severe psychological stress, characteristically one of threatened physical injury or death.

A *fugue state* is a related disorder in which the individual suddenly assumes a new identity (partial or complete), will unexpectedly travel away from his home or area of customary residence, and reports an inability to remember the past.

Depersonalization disorder is the experience of feeling outside of one's body, as if one might be detached from or observing oneself from a vantage point. The feeling that one is in a dream or in some form of suspended animation is common. The patient is not psychotic or delusional, and reality testing remains generally intact. The individual is frequently distressed by this perception and may feel frightened or quite apprehensive that he or she might "lose control and not be able to get it back." Disorders such as panic disorder, schizophrenia, and various forms of epilepsy need to be ruled out when assessing a depersonalization disorder.

Multiple personality disorder occurs when there has been some rather severe early-life physical, sexual, and psychological stress to the patient so as to cause the personality to be fragile. When this occurs, superimposed anxiety can cause a fracturing of the personality into various subunits, with each subunit taking on its own identity. As discussed earlier in the chapter, these identities need not be totally unaware of the existence of other identities or personalities, but for multiple personality to exist, these various personalities need to recurrently take full control of the behavior of the patient. Multiple personalities may be quite intelligent, creative, and insightful individuals. The gradual reintegration of multiple-personality syndrome frequently takes a significant amount of time and must be performed by a professional who has had experience with such disorders.

IV. "The Thought Censoring" Portion of the Mind

Although there is no clear-cut area in the brain where all thoughts are "censored," our mental processes do undergo a censoring phenomenon in which extraneous and irrelevant information is deleted. This allows us to focus on the more pertinent and significant information that we need to address at that moment. This entails the individual having a significant amount of control over his patterns and resultant behaviors at any given time. As with most functions of the mind, when operating in moderation, they are very helpful and contribute to the overall well-being of the individual. However, when out of balance and excessive in degree, then dysfunction and distress can transpire. If anxiety is displaced into this so-called "thought censoring" portion of the mind, one of the more common disorders to be exacerbated is the *obsessive-compulsive disorder*. An individual with this disorder would have recurrent and rather persistent ideas, impulses, or thoughts that are seen as intruding into his consciousness and senses and are generally quite disturbing. For example, an individual might have an obsessive thought "to abandon your faith in God" that seems to intrude into his or her consciousness over and over again, even with the best efforts to suppress or delete this thought. A characteristic of the disorder is a rather involved and rigorous attempt by the individual to suppress or diminish the thoughts or impulses, all the while realizing that these thoughts and impulses are arising from within his or her mind. Compulsions involve the existence of repetitive, purposeful, and often distressful behaviors that are designed to prevent discomfort or neutralize anxiety. The individual will generally recognize that the behavior is excessive and unreasonable, and yet there is a tremendous battle going on within the individual to stop the repetitive behavior. For example, an individual who can't seem to stop washing his hands constantly for fear that there is some dreaded disease or accumulation of dirt on his hands, although rationally he knows that he practices good hygiene and that such extensive and repetitive hand washing is not only unwarranted but is actually causing dryness and irritation to the hands. Well-known men in the church have been afflicted with obsessive-compulsive disorder; for example, the godly John Bunyan who wrote *Grace Abounding to the Chief of Sinners* had the distressing recurring thought of "sell Christ."[8]

In understanding how anxiety can become folded into symptoms as complex as an obsessive-compulsive disorder, it may be helpful to see anxiety as dissectable into three "components." Anxiety 1 is the anxiety that comes from deep within, largely surrounding repressed conflicts and guilt issues dealing with basic self-esteem (injuries sustained in the early developmental years of life). Anxiety 2 is that anxiety emanating from conflicts and perceived threats in everyday living situations. Anxiety 3 comes from confronting some feared object, such as a phobia where there may be fear of elevators, fear of heights, fear of snakes, and so on. Anxiety 3 is frequently dealt with by using desensitization, that is, a form of behavior modification that progressively assists a person in becoming less sensitive and fearful of a perceived frightening object. A common form of behavior modification desensitization performed in our society is to help a child overcome his or her fear of dogs by allowing the child to play with little puppies at a pet store and then slightly older dogs and so forth until the child has overcome any unnatural apprehension of full-grown dogs. Anxiety 2 is generally dealt with by counselors helping a person solve present-day situational problems with commonsense endeavors. Many pastoral and religious counselors deal extensively with the priorities and life-style issues that surface surrounding Anxiety 2. Anxiety 1 is that deeper anxiety that is frequently dealt with by extensive counseling, including psychoanalytic configuration. This seeks to apply scriptural truths and healing at the basic roots of certain deep-seated problems producing Anxiety 1. The following is an example of an obsessive-compulsive disorder and the types of anxiety that were noted to be contributing to the disorder in this young man.

CASE STUDY: Tom was a thirty-year-old white male who came for an appointment because he was depressed. Several precipitating causes (financial problems, business problems, religious confusion) were discussed. However, the really interesting dynamics to this case came out when the patient discussed his past.

He described his parents as very strict disciplinarians. When he was young, his parents would spank him at times, and at other times wash out his mouth with soap. While still in grade school, he developed the compulsion to wash his hands. He would wash his hands repeatedly and would avoid touching things so his hands would not get dirty. Because of these symptoms, the parents consulted a child psychologist, who suggested that the parents not be so hard on him. They took his advice and the symptoms largely disappeared. However, even today, he said he would wash things often, wrap food several times, and is very perfectionistic.

The dynamics of the case could be explained as follows:

Stressful early-life situation (domineering parents)

↓

Anxiety produced

↓

Anxiety repressed into subconscious (which can be called Anxiety 1)

↓

Stressful current-day situation arises (financial and business pressures)

↓

Anxiety produced (which can be called Anxiety 2)

↓

Anxiety 1 also aroused

↓

Anxiety displaced to compulsive action (i.e., obsessive-compulsive disorder)

↓

Anxiety 1 also aroused by Anxiety 2

In this case, Anxiety 1 and Anxiety 2 needed to be dealt with by the patient. With psychotherapy, the patient began to let up on himself, relax more, fret less, and be less serious. As he began to improve, so did his confusion over Christianity. He began to stop blaming God for his depression. He began to realize God was not trying to punish him. He stopped reading so many religious books for answers and turned to the Word for spiritual nourishment.

The following are examples of cases of obsessive-compulsive disorder told from the psychiatrist's viewpoint.

CASE STUDY: Dora was a twenty-year-old lady who came to me complaining of depression. However, the psychiatric interview revealed there was much more involved than just depression. Dora felt she must repeatedly ask God to forgive her for every moment-to-moment bad thought or action. She had become immobilized. She even doubted the sincerity of her request for forgiveness and would then have to ask God to forgive her for that. Her daily quiet times had turned from worship to hours of inward introspection. On one occasion, Dora felt the compulsion to curse over the phone and did so. This was the last thing she consciously wanted to do, and she felt very grieved. Her symptoms had even gone to the point that she thought she heard voices on one occasion. She was profoundly depressed and was near overt psychosis. Her diagnosis was *obsessive-compulsive disorder*.

Recognizing the patient had three problems (physical, psychological, and spiritual), I started therapy. First, through medication, I began to attack the biochemical abnormalities present. As the patient's physiology returned to normal, she started to make progress. I also instructed her to limit her devotional time to five minutes per day for the time being. She was reminded that this was for worship, not introspection. She was encouraged in therapy to be less rigid, less serious, and less introspective. The last time I saw her, she had adjusted and was doing very well. She was still a very dedicated Christian, but now she had balance.

CASE STUDY: Caroline was a very dedicated Christian girl. She came for an appointment because she wanted guidance about a spiritual issue.

She felt compelled to make apologies to everyone. She would apologize for the least little matter. This was beginning to get her into trouble in certain areas. For example, she was a nursing student, and when she kept apologizing to a teacher for not reading every word of an assignment, he became angry with her. Rigidity and perfectionism characterized every aspect of Caroline's life. Through therapy, she was able to begin to see this and even laugh at it a little. She seemed a little shocked when I told her I felt that her feeling so guilty over any mistake or fault was more a matter of pride than humility. Someone would have to be almost omnipotent to cause the reverberations she felt she caused with the slightest error. Through therapy, she was able to begin to see that the real issue was not the compulsion to confess, but that this was only a symptom of some deeper subconscious anxiety. In other words, in an attempt to control some subconscious anxiety, she had displaced it from its original source to the compulsion to confess. She began to relax more, have more fun, become more involved with other young people at church, and to steadily improve.

CASE STUDY: Beth, a twenty-five-year-old white female, came to see me because of guilt feelings. She felt guilty about everything. She felt guilty over a minor scratch she might cause to a car. She felt guilty for leaving a dripping faucet on. She felt guilty about throwing away a tissue paper for fear it might have contained a contact lens. She felt guilty for a college teacher's giving her a grade that was too high.

She also worried about her hands being dirty after touching a doorknob. She worried about making some mistake at her job that would cost the company money. All of these traits are *obsessive-compulsive.*

As with hysterical neurosis and schizophrenia, people through the years have often been quick to say that an individual with an *obsessive-compulsive* problem is demon-possessed. Thus, a few words on demon possession may be useful at this point. There is today an upsurge of interest in the topic of demon possession. Prominent magazines have had feature articles dealing with the occult. The film *The Exorcist* was among the top films in amount of money grossed. Young people, not finding solutions to their problems, are turning to the supernatural.

On the one hand, I believe the occult is a mark of our age. On the other hand, much of what is suspected to be demon possession could be one of several psychiatric problems—acute manic psychosis, obsessive-compulsive disorder, multiple-personality

disorder, temporal lobe epilepsy, and schizophrenia. Because of
the current interest in demon possession, much confusion will
result, not unsimilar to the widespread confusion that existed in
the fifteenth century when the *Malleus Maleficarum* was written
to help in the diagnosis of witches and demon possession. Unstable individuals, impressionable and hysterical personalities,
and borderline schizophrenics could believe they were demon-
possessed after watching films that focus intensely on demonic
possession.

Safety for the Christian is not found in being overly interested
in demon possession but in having a renewed interest in Christ
our Lord. Because of the confusion of our day, only a living
knowledge of God's Word will give stability. The pursuit of God,
God's Word, prayer, and fellowship with godly people—these
are the solutions.

Another disorder of the "thought censoring" or information-
processing function of the mind is *attention deficit disorder.*
Attention deficit disorder, previously known as hyperactivity or
hyperkinesis, is a disorder that surfaces largely in the preado-
lescent years and affects a youngster's ability to appropriately
concentrate on and pay attention to his or her environment. In
essence, these youngsters cannot censor out extraneous information and remain in a state of alertness and calmness while
they attend to information learning or carrying out structured
tasks. Attention deficit disorder occurs in as many as 3 percent
of children and is six to nine times more common in males than
in females.[9] A child with attention deficit disorder will frequently have six months of several of the following symptoms:
being easily distracted by external stimuli, difficulty waiting his
or her turn in line for games or group situations, difficulty sustaining attention tasks, difficulty playing quietly, frequently talking excessively, or having problems remaining seated when told
to do so. The child may also fidget or squirm when trying to sit
still and frequently interrupts others, becoming intrusive in
other children's conversations or games. Such youngsters appear
to not be listening to what is being said to them, and they may
have difficulty with their schoolwork. They may race through
their homework without adequately completing it or sit for long

periods of time in front of their work without purposefully accomplishing it while their minds drift from subject to subject. The youngster may focus on all kinds of minor distractions away from the task at hand. The onset is usually before the age of seven, and the child frequently has a normal level of intelligence. The child may have a learning disorder as well and may learn significantly more efficiently through one sensory input (for example, hearing information spoken) than through another sensory input (note taking). Some of these children also have some "soft neurological signs" such as problems with poor hand-eye coordination. Parents of children with attention deficit disorder are often well-meaning and highly involved individuals who may come to the counselor frustrated and emotionally burned out. They may describe the youngster as having a "perpetual running motor" and may have been told by school and church teachers that the child is difficult to control. Although he does not appear to be intentionally mischievous, he seems never to be able to follow instructions properly and will not finish assigned tasks. He appears to be perpetually disrupting the order and the function of the classroom, and his work is often messy and performed impulsively and haphazardly. He tends to interrupt his classmates, blurting out phrases and frequently provoking the ire of his peers. In evaluating the child with attention deficit disorder, oppositional defiant or conduct disorder would need to be ruled out. Also a possibility is that, through problematic behaviors, the child is simply expressing anxiety arising from parental conflicts at home, sibling discord, or conflicts within his or her peer group at school, church, or in the neighborhood.

V. Anxiety Displaced to a Neutral Object

When anxiety levels build and are displaced or transferred onto a neutral object (such as fear of snakes, heights, elevators, etc.), this is referred to as a *phobia*. A *simple phobia* is a disorder in which there is an unwarranted and persistent fear of a particular and well-defined stimulus (fear of having panic attacks is considered a panic disorder and has been described previously in this chapter). The individual with a simple phobia can have an extreme fear of what would otherwise appear to be common-place in daily living. The individual may recognize the absurdity of his or her fear but cannot help the fear and is not under direct conscious control.

The dynamics of a simple phobia could be explained as follows:

Stressful early-life situations
↓
Anxiety produced
↓
Anxiety repressed into subconscious (which can be called Anxiety 1)
↓
Stressful current-day situation arises, producing Anxiety 2
↓
Anxiety displaced to phobia (fear of elevators, heights, etc.)
↓
Anxiety produced, secondary to worrying over the phobia (which can be called Anxiety 3)—individual attempts to control Anxiety 1 and Anxiety 2 with the phobia which produces Anxiety 3

Actually, then, the three levels of anxiety must be dealt with in counseling. Some schools (behavior modification) deal mainly with Anxiety 3 and help the person to overcome his irrational fear through desensitization. Other schools (some religious counselors) deal mainly with Anxiety 2, helping the person to deal with the present-day situational problem. And yet other schools (psychoanalytic) deal mainly with Anxiety 1.

Perhaps this can be more clearly seen in the obsessive-compulsive neurotic who fears committing the unpardonable sin. Again, all three levels of anxiety must be dealt with in counseling. Certainly, the subject's intense Anxiety 3 of committing the unpardonable sin must be dealt with by the use of Scriptures. The counselee also needs help with Anxiety 2 and his present-day situational problem. Finally, Anxiety 1 and the early childhood fears must be handled.

A *social phobia* involves an individual's fear of social situations. The individual dreads that he will commit some act that is humiliating or embarrassing. Although the individual may recognize that the fear is excessive and unreasonable, the urge to avoid social situations and the anxiety associated with those situations is nevertheless quite intense. Such need to avoid social situations may interfere with the individual's occupational performance and cause a lot of embarrassment.

Agoraphobia is essentially a fear of being in places where an individual feels vulnerable or somehow exposed. The individual may especially have this fear when the situation carries with it a dread that escape or avoidance of the situation might be quite difficult or embarrassing. Individuals with agoraphobia may progressively isolate themselves from social situations; they may stop going to church and visiting friends in the neighborhood and then gradually reach a position where they do not want to leave their home. In severe cases, they can reach a point where they are frightened even to leave a particular room in a home. Such individuals may require a companion when trying to travel away from home and can develop intense anxiety. Panic attacks are not uncommonly associated with agoraphobia. Usually agoraphobia onsets in the twenties or thirties and it may persist for years. It is far more common in females than in males.

VI. The "Addictive Zone" of the Mind

When anxiety occurs and is subsequently displaced into the so-called addictive zone of the mind, then various dependencies and addictions can develop. These addictions may vary from dependencies on drugs and alcohol to addictions related to foods such as morbid obesity, bulimia, and anorexia. An individual with *anorexia nervosa* manifests a reluctance to maintain a body weight over the absolute minimum for healthy functioning and then maintains a body weight usually at least 15 percent below the expected norms for their height, age, and bone frame. They have an intense fear of gaining weight and frequently wear baggy clothing to disguise their actual body configuration. Distortions of their body shape are common. For example, anoretic females, when asked to draw a configuration of their own body, will draw themselves as quite obese when in fact they are emaciated. They may

develop fixations on a certain area of their body as being "too fat."
For example, anoretic females can look as if they had been in a
concentration camp due to their self-starvation yet sit in a chair
and poke their widened little thigh muscle saying, "see there, see
that fat, it's too gross." Also, females will frequently cease men-
struating when they have anorexia. It is a very severe disorder
with a mortality rate of between 5 and 18 percent. Severe weight
loss often necessitates hospitalization to prevent death from star-
vation. The disorder frequently onsets in the late adolescence or
early twenties and is predominant in females (95 percent).[10]

Bulimia is also a severe eating disorder that involves recurring
episodes of excessive consumption of large amounts of food in a
circumscribed period of time with lack of control over the eating
behavior. These individuals will then self-induce vomiting or
use laxatives or diuretics to purge themselves of the food they
have eaten. Bulimia is also largely seen in females rather than
males. To qualify as a bulimic disorder, there needs to be a
minimum average of two binge-eating episodes weekly for a
period of at least three months. There is also an associated over-
concern with body weight and shape. In our experience, individuals with true bulimia have a high incidence of sexual abuse
in their developmental years.

Pica is another eating disorder, seen in the early developmental years, which needs to be distinguished from autism or schizophrenia (pervasive developmental disorder of childhood) or
Kleine-Levin syndrome. Children with pica will persistently eat
substances that are nonnutritive such as plaster, string, paint,
hair, leaves, insects, pebbles, and so on. The child has no aversion to food. Pica will usually subside in early childhood but may
persist into adolescence. It is very rare in adulthood. In a true
case of pica, mental retardation would need to be ruled out as a
coexistent diagnostic consideration.

As anxiety finds areas for displacement within the personality,
then other areas of function may be adversely affected. For example, sexual disorders such as *paraphilia* can have a very addictive nature. These can include exhibitionism, fetishism,
pedophilia, sexual masochism, sexual sadism, transvestite fetishism, and voyeurism. The treatment of sexual addictions has

gained much understanding during the last several years largely through the work of Patrick Karnes, author of the book *Out of the Shadows*, which deals with approaching sexual addictions through Twelve-Step recovery work, much the same as is used in helping recovering alcoholics or drug addicts. Unfortunately, those with sexual addictions have for years felt ashamed and humiliated by their disorder to the point that they would rarely seek professional help, carrying on their disorders in painful seclusion with little means for therapeutic assistance.

Another form of addiction that is now being better understood is *relationship addiction or co-dependency*. Individuals who are dealing with anxiety, especially during the early developmental years when patterns of relationships are being established, may be drawn toward establishing co-dependent relationships with others. Co-dependent relationships can be quite powerful in their compulsive hold on individuals. There is a rapidly growing body of information on understanding how the addiction to certain interpersonal relationships (co-dependency) can place an individual in a great deal of bondage. The co-dependent individual frequently comes from a dysfunctional family and may well be actively involved in church and community activities. Co-dependent individuals, however, may pay a high personal price of painful consequences of their feeling addicted to relationships to other individuals. Many times they no longer feel that they have an independent identity in and of themselves, and they may labor under the constant fear that they will be rejected and abandoned by others. In the book, *Love Is Choice, Recovery for Co-Dependent Relationships*, Drs. Hemfelt, Minirth, and Meier define *co-dependency* as "an addiction of people, behaviors or things." Co-dependency is the fallacy of trying to control interior feelings by controlling people, things, and events on the outside. To the co-dependent, control or the lack of it is central to every aspect of life.[11] Drs. Hemfelt, Minirth, and Meier describe what they call the "ten traits of a co-dependent" as follows:

1. A co-dependent is driven by one or more compulsions. (Workaholism is one particular compulsion in which co-dependents are frequently highly engaged. The intense in-

vestment in work to the exclusion of other priorities, drive, and the drive for that work to meet a variety of intense needs such as self-esteem, achievement, satisfaction, worth, affiliations with others, and approval from God may indicate workaholism. Although outwardly an "acceptable" addiction, workaholism has destroyed the lives of many individuals and their families. We suggest *The Workaholic and His Family* by Paul Meier as good reading on this subject.)

2. The co-dependent is bound and often tormented by the way things were in the dysfunctional family of origin.
3. The co-dependent's self-esteem (and frequently maturity) is very low.
4. A co-dependent is certain his or her happiness hinges on others.
5. Conversely, a co-dependent feels inordinately responsible for others.
6. The co-dependent's relationship with a spouse or significant other person is marred by a damaging, unstable lack of balance between dependence and independence.
7. A co-dependent is a master of denial and repression.
8. The co-dependent worries about things he or she can't change but may well try to change them.
9. A co-dependent's life is punctuated by extremes.
10. A co-dependent is constantly looking for the something that is missing or lacking in life.[12]

Other addictive behaviors that can be seen as a means of displacing otherwise intolerable anxiety are chronic pathologic gambling, persistent involvement in extensive risk-taking behaviors, and kleptomania. Other usual behaviors that border on being addictive in nature, are repetitive, and are difficult to treat are pyromania (the deliberate and willful setting of fires on more than one occasion, a sense of tension and arousal prior to setting the fires, and intense pleasure and gratification when the fire is set) and trichotillomania (a disorder characterized by recurrent failure to cease and desist from impulses to pull out one's own hair). As mentioned above, a major form of addictive behavior involves the abuse of alcohol or drugs. The diagnosis and proper treatment of alcoholism or chemical abuse is a complex area. The best treatment programs at this point involve a mixture of spiritual awareness with solid work in the Twelve-Step approach to recovery from chemical dependence. Two books that are Christian in orientation and deal with the field of substance abuse in a comprehensive fashion are *Counselling for Substance Abuse and Addiction*, by Steve Van Cleave, M.D., Walter Byrd, M.D., and Kathy Revell, R.N., and *Taking Control*, Frank Minirth, M.D., et al.

VII. The Self-Concept or Self-Identity Area of the Mind

When anxiety, either chronic or acute in nature, is displaced into the self-concept or self-identity area of the mind, then the individual's sense of personal integrity and self-worth may be compromised. If a situation occurs that suddenly thrusts upon the individual an overwhelming amount of anxiety or distress, then an *adjustment disorder* may develop. Adjustment disorders are essentially a maladaptive reaction to a psychosocial stressor (or several stressors) that has predated the onset of the adjustment disorder by no more than three months. The disorder should not have been persisting for more than six months. The symptoms of the maladaptive reaction are generally in excess of the normal and expected reaction to the stressors, and there is discernible impairment in an individual's ability to function at home, at work, in the community, at church, and so on.

Adjustment disorders are of various types. They include adjustment disorder with depressed mood where the predominant manifestation is tearfulness, sadness, feelings of hopelessness, and a depressed mood. There is also an adjustment disorder with a conduct disturbance in which the individual may show disruptive and excessive behavior quite out of context for his usual demeanor (such as reckless driving, fighting, shirking legal responsibilities, truancy). There is also an adjustment disorder with physical complaints such as headaches, backaches, fatigue, and so forth, that is not diagnosable as coming from a specific physical cause. An adjustment disorder with an anxious mood is an adjustment disorder that predominantly portrays itself with symptoms of restlessness, jitteriness, worry, and usually dread about some event or situation.

Adjustment disorders can cause social withdrawal from others, especially from social situations that were normally enjoyable such as church or civic activities. Problems with work or academic functioning in an individual whose previous performance at work or school was adequate may be manifested as an inhibition.

If anxiety is chronically, over a long period of time, displaced into the self-concept or self-identity area of the mind, then intensely *negative self-talk* may develop. Negative self-talk involves the individual's developing a series of "lies" or deceptions about his own worth, dignity as a person, or value to himself or God. Irrational beliefs about one's self serve to undermine and distort the individual's belief in his own worth or suitableness as a person and can erode the person's level of function to the point where he develops a significant depression. The concept of *depression* (including manic depressive illness) will be dealt with in depth in chapter 7. When dealing with an individual, however, who is struggling with some fairly straightforward issue of self-worth and self-esteem, the following seven practical ideas may be helpful in assisting that person to foster a healthier self-concept.

1. Allow for flaws or imperfections in your behavior; don't focus on your negatives.
2. Commit to praise yourself for a solid effort and seek to see mistakes as opportunities to learn.
3. Set realistic goals, and give yourself credit for partial success toward your goals.
4. Don't exaggerate the negatives in situations; avoid "awfulizing" or "catastrophizing."
5. Gather and use resources in your environment to work for you.
6. Share with others (in whom you have confidence) accomplishments, realistic appraisals of yourself, and your honest feelings in dealing with life's obstacles.
7. Endorse and compliment others on their achievements others will be likely to treat you in a like manner.

As we are looking over the rather broad amount of information that has been presented in this chapter, it may be helpful to present an overview of how various factors can combine to cause psychological problems.

Factors Causing Psychological Problems

There are several important factors in the development of a mental illness.[13] These factors and the various forms of the development of mental illness are diagramed below:

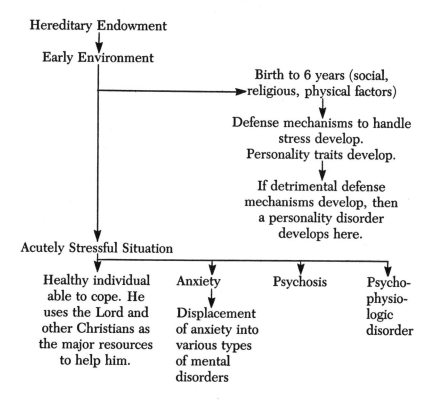

Hereditary Endowment

Early Environment

Birth to 6 years (social, religious, physical factors)

Defense mechanisms to handle stress develop.
Personality traits develop.

If detrimental defense mechanisms develop, then a personality disorder develops here.

Acutely Stressful Situation

| Healthy individual able to cope. He uses the Lord and other Christians as the major resources to help him. | Anxiety ↓ Displacement of anxiety into various types of mental disorders | Psychosis | Psycho-physio-logic disorder |

A book could be written on the importance of each one of the diagramed factors in the development of mental illness. Mental illness is not so simple and often is not caused by one factor alone A spiritual problem may be the cause of the emotional problem, but other factors often come into play or are responsible.

For example, the genetic background is important when examining a mental problem. We have seen one mental problem in particular, *manic-depressive psychosis,* where an unusually high proportion of the relatives had also had the problem. And, as stated elsewhere in other chapters, scientific studies have documented that children of schizophrenic parents develop schizophrenia significantly more often than other children, even when they are raised away from the parents.[14] Furthermore, one does not have to look far to see that personality traits run in families. Just as dogs pass on personality traits (German shepherd—aggressive, St. Bernard—friendly), so do humans.

Second, the importance of environmental background has probably been overstated through the past several years. However, there is no doubt that this factor is of much importance in forming a personality. Children are taught to be humble, aggressive, polite, or rude. We have seen parents who wonder why their sixteen-year-old Johnny is rude, rebellious, and disobedient, yet the parents have never disciplined him. Physical health could also be included in this category. Children or adults who are physically ill often have less capacity to withstand emotional stress.

Usually, a third factor is necessary for a psychological problem to develop. This third factor is a precipitating stress. Although one may have hereditary factors present and may have had a difficult early environment, a psychological disorder may never develop unless he is in an acutely stressful situation.

Truly, the genetic and environmental backgrounds are factors of major importance. To deny this is naive. However, it is equally naive to use these as excuses for present conduct. Many problems are brought about through irresponsible behavior. What Apostle Paul said many years ago is still true: ". . . whatsoever a man soweth, that shall he also reap" (Galatians 6:7). Many times emotional problems are brought about through irresponsible behavior, sins, just not knowing, or failing to rely on the resources that a Christian has at his disposal.

The counselor needs certain criteria by which to reach conclusions concerning the counselee and his personality trends.

THE AUTHORS

5 The Evaluative Workup

Every psychiatrist, minister, psychologist, or counselor will follow different procedures for obtaining the background information necessary to help the patient. The following is an evaluation sequence that we typically use in the Minirth-Meier Clinic system in assessing a new patient. The format is a standard one used commonly in psychiatric training programs.[1]

May we submit our knowledge to the guidance of God and pray that what we discover can be used to help the counselee to grow in Christ.

Circumstances of Referral and Presenting Problem

This is simply a statement of who the counselee is and a brief statement usually in the counselee's own words of what he understands his problem to be. An example would be: "This twenty-four-year-old white male from Jonesboro, Arkansas, was referred to me by his minister, Reverend John Ward. The patient's chief complaint was 'depression.' "

History of Present Problem

Under this heading, the counselor goes into more detail about the presenting problem. The counselor will need to know when the problem first started, if there were previous episodes, the duration of the episodes, what helped to relieve them, who was previously sought as a counselor, what medication was used, and what event, if any, precipitated the problem most recently. In addition, current symptoms that are present and the severity of these symptoms are very important. Also, the counselor will need to know the current events contributing to the problem and how the counselee has attempted to deal with these events and his problems.

Past History

A past history often reveals significant data that aid in understanding and helping the counselee. While the focus is not on the past, the counselor would be omitting significant data to ignore the past entirely.

First, data concerning the counselee's birth and early development should be considered. Data obtained here can reveal insight into the cause of a learning disability, mental retardation, and other mental problems. The nature and duration of the mother's pregnancy, the birth weight, complications at birth, the age when walking and talking began, and the living situation at the time of birth are all significant.

Second, data relating to the family can be very helpful. The counselor will need to know the parents' age, health, current residency, and, most importantly, a description of each of their personalities. The relationship the counselee had with each parent is also very important. Not only are data relating to the parents helpful, but data relating to siblings are helpful, also. The number of siblings, the relationship with the siblings, and the order of birth are all important. From this kind of data, the counselor can learn much about the counselee's personality, about how he relates, and even about how he may view God inasmuch as we tend to view God as we view our genetic parents.

Third, the events that occurred during school should be considered. What kind of grades did the counselee make? How much study did this require? Did he have many surface friendships or a few close ones? What were his main interests? When did the counselee start dating? Did he graduate from high school? And if so, when? Did he attend college? What were the major events that happened during the college years? From such data, the counselor can be alerted to such factors as underachievement or overachievement tendencies. This may explain why he has tension at his job. Also, from such data, the counselor can determine how the counselee relates to people. He can note whether the counselee's educational level and functional level correlate

Fourth, there are several other areas about which the counselor will need data. Was the counselee in the military service and, if so, what type of discharge did he receive? What is the counselee's occupation? Does he have a history of changing jobs frequently? How many times has he been married? What does the patient list as the causes for any previous divorces? Is the counselee's spouse in good health? How do they relate? How are they compatible? How are they different? Does the counselee have children? How old are they? Are they in good health? Does the counselee have a history of drug abuse? Does he have a history of conflicts with the law? From such data, the counselor can learn about the emotional stability of the counselee in general. He can learn if he has sociopathic tendencies. He can learn about various stress factors heretofore not discussed.

Finally, a history of the counselee's relationship to Christ is very important. Has the counselee accepted Christ as his Savior? Does he know how one becomes a Christian? How has he grown spiritually through the years? What does he do for spiritual growth now? Would his strongest area be Christian fellowship, Bible study, prayer, or witnessing for Christ? In which of these four areas does he need to grow most?

Evaluative Examination

The first parameter in an evaluative examination is *general appearance.* Does the counselee appear to be his stated age? What is his demeanor? Is he tense, suspicious, grave, slouchy, dignified, manneristic, or gracious? What is the condition of his clothes? What is his general behavior: Is he restless? Is there any strange or unusual behavior present? The answers to these questions determine much.

If a counselee appears older than his stated age, he may have spent many years obsessively worrying. When he appears many years younger, with few, if any, wrinkles, he may be a schizophrenic, for he may have escaped anxiety through the years by escaping reality. If the counselee appears suspicious, he may have paranoid tendencies. Noting that a counselee is meticulously dressed gives a clue that he may have obsessive-compulsive tendencies, and thus guilt may be one of his problems. If the counselee is rather unkempt, he may be depressed. When depressed, men stop shaving, and women stop fixing their hair and putting on makeup. If the counselee is obese, he may be depressed and is compensating by overeating. When the counselee is seductive in dress and action, a hysterical trend exists and also, perhaps, immaturity. When the counselee has grease on several areas of his tie, he may have an organic brain syndrome inasmuch as most people would rid themselves of such a tie. If the patient shows unusual behavior, he may be psychotic. For example, he may keep looking around as though he is hearing or seeing something. If he is restless, overt anxiety is present for some reason. Observing that a counselee will not look up and holds his head down alerts the counselor to think of depression. Whether the counselee's greeting is vigorous, seductive, or warm tells much. If the counselee has a history of much antisocial behavior, but the therapist is drawn to like him, he may be a sociopath. When the counselee steps into the office and does not close the door or is late for the appointment, he may have passive-aggressive tendencies.

If the counselee is an adolescent, the counselor should be cautious about making an official psychiatric diagnosis since the normal adolescent *is* abnormal! To be sure, adolescence is a time of many adjustment reactions that present in many ways.

If the counselee is a young child, the counselor will want to know the relationship with the mother. If the child is in the age range of four to twelve, the counselor will especially focus on the parent of the same sex, since the child is at a stage of introjecting into his personality the attitudes of his parents, especially the one of like sex.

When the counselee is in his fifties or sixties, has always been very productive and conscientious, but has suddenly become depressed, the counselor thinks of an involutional melancholic process seen often at this age. In the old, the counselor is especially apt to look for organic causes.

In counselees with physical problems, the counselor should be aware of possible depression. If the counselee appears shy, aloof, and introverted, the counselor may think of schizoid trends. If he demonstrates low frustration tolerance and an outburst of verbal abuse, the counselor has clues to explosive trends that are present and poorly controlled. When the counselee presents himself as a result of marked anxiety at work and the counselor notes ineffectual responses to questions, the counselor will consider that the counselee is producing beyond his capabilities and thus frustration is resulting.

Some of the above parameters are picked up by evaluation of general appearance and can be helpful in determining the personality trends and, thus, potential problems of the counselee.

The second parameter in a mental examination is *intellectual proficiency*. Is the counselee oriented to time, place, and person? How many digits can he recall immediately after they are presented to him? Six to seven forward is average. How is his memory of both recent and remote events? How is his knowledge of general information compared to his educational background? Can the counselee subtract serial sevens from one hundred; can he divide one hundred by seven? Has he had any periods of amnesia?

These questions indicate whether an individual has an organic brain syndrome. This would be important in evaluating the aged. They provide clues as to whether he could concentrate or was preoccupied with other thoughts as in depression. They would indicate roughly his I.Q. and thus give valuable information concerning overachievers.

The third parameter is *communication*. What is the rate of conversation? Is the conversation logical or does the counselee ramble? Is the conversation relevant? Can the counselor follow the train of conversation of the counselee or are there loose associations present? Is the conversation spontaneous or resistant? Does the thought content make sense? Can he interpret proverbs, demonstrating he is capable of abstract thinking? Does the counselee have an obsession or preoccupation? Has he ever heard voices?

If the counselor cannot follow the conversation of a counselee, but rather the associations are loose and the counselee cannot interpret a simple proverb as "Don't cross a bridge until you get to it" and he reports hearing voices, the counselor may strongly suspect schizophrenia. If the counselee cannot rid himself of thoughts that are foreign to his usual thinking, he may be obsessive-compulsive. If the counselee has had periods of amnesia, this may be a type of hysterical symptom. If the counselee speaks spontaneously, he tends to be extroverted. On the other hand, he may only answer questions, a tendency indicative of being introverted.

The fourth parameter that an evaluative examination includes is *mood*. How does the counselee describe his mood? Does he say he is happy, sad, or indifferent? Does the counselee cry often? What is his facial expression? Is his expression consistent with the way he describes his feelings? Has the counselee made any suicidal gestures? Has he ever felt like life was just not worth living? How is the counselee sleeping and eating? If he is married, what is the sexual relationship between him and his spouse?

A counselee may describe his mood accurately or he may not; therefore, other parameters are important. For example, a depressed person may have trouble going to sleep, or he may awaken in the early morning hours. His appetite is usually poor. If the counselee has made several unsuccessful suicidal gestures, he may be hysterical rather than depressed. Thus, the counseling would be totally different. An individual may have a flat affect. If so, depression or even schizophrenia is a consideration.

I hope the above criteria are helpful, but they must not be overread. The evaluative examination depends on many factors and a life history of how a person functions socially and biologically.

The Impression

This is simply a statement of what the counselor feels the real problem is. It is usually very short, such as *depression, adjustment reaction,* or any one of numerous descriptions.

Dynamic Formulation

In the dynamic formulation, however, the counselor attempts to integrate all he has learned about the patient (hereditary factors, environmental factors, basic personality type, defense mechanisms, religious history, and precipitating events) into a cohesive explanation of how the counselee has evolved up to the present. An example would be the following hypothetical case of John Doe, a *manic-depressive.*

"Hereditary factors do seem to be important in this case. Three of John's relatives have also suffered from *manic-depressive* problems. However, early environmental factors cannot be ignored, as reference to past history has proved. In short, hereditary factors combine with early environmental factors to produce detrimental defense mechanisms and ways of coping. When John was subjected to increased stress last year with the death of his father, he decompensated into a *manic-depressive* episode. Since that time, John was led to Christ by a friend. He has become involved in a local church and is now beginning to cope well."

What follows is an outline of a typical evaluative workup:

The Evaluative Workup

    I. Presenting Situation
   II. History of Present Problem
 III. Past History
 IV. Evaluative Examination
   V. Clinical Impression
 VI. Tentative Dynamic Formulation
VII. Initial Counseling Plan

———————————————————

Signature

"Though I say, 'I will forget my complaint, I will leave off my *sad* countenance, and be cheerful,' I am afraid
of all my pains."

JOB 9:27, 28 NAS

6 Physical Condition and Emotional Problems

The Whole-Person Concept

A counselor is responsible for considering more than the surface
mental or emotional problem that an individual presents. Man
consists of a body, soul, and spirit, and each must be considered.
Physical disease and problems may affect the mental capacities
of a person and produce emotional problems. Likewise, spiritual
problems can affect the mental functioning of an individual and
produce emotional problems.

Related Problems

First, a person's physical condition should be considered in
any apparent emotional disorder, whether it pertains to mild
depression or psychosis. For example, early in Dr. Minirth's
residency in psychiatry, he was assigned to manage a lady who
was overtly psychotic. He greeted her and then listened as she
rambled on in religious jargon. Her speech was rapid, and she
seemed "high." Judging from previous cases of *manic-depressive
psychosis* and his impression, he concluded that she fit this con
dition. In short, an individual with the manic phase of *manic-
depressive psychosis* would be apt to have extreme elation, flight
of ideas, pressure of speech, impaired judgment, and delusions.

128

The delusions may center around religious or sexual preoccupations. Later, in the course of discussion, a relative revealed that the patient had been treating herself for nervousness with an over-the-counter medication. This particular medication was prone to produce these symptoms when taken in excess. After several days, the patient had eliminated the medication from her system, and her symptoms cleared.

Hyperactivity in children is another example of an apparent emotional problem that may really be physical. There is a neurological impairment that results in hyperactivity. If not placed on medication, however, secondary emotional problems may develop. When placed on appropriate medication, the hyperactivity decreases, and the child is able to sit still and concentrate as other children do. The hyperactivity is not the result of an emotional problem of the child nor of inadequate child care by the parents. It should be mentioned that all cases diagnosed as "hyperactive" are not always hyperactive because of physical causes; therefore, emotional causes may need to be sought. Definite neurological signs and other factors must be considered in making a correct diagnosis

CASE STUDY: John was a typical example of a hyperactive child. He could not sit still in school, had a short attention span, and poor concentration. John was considered a "bad" boy and a troublemaker.

I saw John and found him to have moderate signs in a neurological examination. The rest of the evaluation also confirmed the diagnosis of a neurologically based hyperactivity problem. John was started on medication and the teachers quickly noted the change. John began to pay attention in class. His concentration improved. He was not so disruptive.

Educators are being alerted to this problem, and today these children are often recognized and thus referred for help. Such was not the case until recently.

Schizophrenia is another example of an emotional problem that may have a physical base. Children may also be schizophrenic or autistic since infancy. This would indicate again a primary biochemical or physical problem. Children with a schizophrenic family heritage are more apt to develop schizophrenia than the average child. Even when raised apart from his genetic family, a child of schizophrenic parents still has a significantly higher chance of developing schizophrenia than the rest of the population. Again, this indicates that physical factors are important.

Hypoglycemia is another condition that may cause nervousness or even a marked change in personality. This may result in diabetes mellitus from an overdose of insulin or insulin-releasing agent. It also may result from an organic cause or it could be functional. If the cause is simply functional, which is often the case, the problem can be helped by relieving stressful situations, eating more often, and eating more protein than carbohydrates.

Although hypoglycemia does exist, we would point out that it has tended to be overemphasized among Christians as a cause of emotional problems. However, certainly some individuals have reduced their moodiness and nervousness through a healthier diet and the consumption of less refined sugar.

Hypothyroidism and *hyperthyroidism* are glandular physical problems that may manifest emotional disorders causing nervousness.[1] Hence, the hyperthyroid patient may appear as a thin, excitable, nervous person. Mental symptoms vary from exhilaration to severe depression. In contrast, the hypothyroid patient may appear overweight and slow, but also nervous. In either case, with proper treatment both improve greatly.

Among the many physical diseases also carrying an emotional component is *mononucleosis*. It is well known that individuals suffering from this may develop depression.

CASE STUDY. Harry was such a case. He had been a good student for two years in medical school. He then developed mononucleosis. After he recovered, he suffered from depression and for a while had a difficult time with his grades.

Physical Stress is a physical problem that results in psychological problems. It is not as rare as the above, but a condition common to most at some time. Physical exhaustion may beget or accentuate emotional problems. Christ Himself knew the importance of rest after a hard day of work (*see* Mark 4:38).

In the discussion of physical problems causing emotional symptoms, one more condition deserves comment because of its prevalence during old age. This is the problem of *organic brain syndrome*, which ranges from very mild to severe in advanced years. Because of such physical factors as increased arteriosclerosis in the brain, or *Alzheimer's disease*, these individuals are more emotionally labile, less flexible in their opinions, and may lose some of their usual restraints. Also, undesirable personality traits may become more prominent. Individuals having this syndrome manifest *accentuation* of basic personality traits and *release* of previous inhibitions. Of course, these individuals need more patience from others.

In summary, almost any physical problem can accentuate emotional problems. The ability to cope with daily stresses is greatly decreased in physical illness. Thus, the hyperactive child will be much less likely to develop secondary emotional problems if on medication. The diabetic in good control will avoid unnecessary conflicts, as will individuals with hypothyroidism, hyperthyroidism, or anemia.

Why art thou cast down, O my soul?
and why art thou disquieted within
me? hope thou in God: for I shall yet
praise him, who is the health of my
countenance, and my God.

PSALM 43:5

7   Depression

Dr. Minirth recounts the following vignette from his office practice in Richardson, Texas:

> The secretary came to my office door and told me there was a patient waiting to see me. I went to the door and asked the patient to come into my office. A lady with a sad facial expression was sitting in a wheelchair, and her sister and cousin were present. The sister wheeled the patient into my office.
>
> Discussion soon revealed that the patient wasn't sleeping nights, had no appetite, and was crying much of the time. She had also attempted suicide the night before.
>
> At one point in the conversation I asked, "Do you know why you are depressed?"
>
> "I don't know," was the answer as she burst into tears.
>
> "How long have you been depressed?" I asked.
>
> Her sister interrupted, "May I speak?"
>
> "Sure," I replied.
>
> Her sister continued, "For about the past month, she has been very depressed."
>
> "Did something happen a month ago?" I asked.
>
> "No," her sister answered.
>
> The patient appeared psychotically depressed so I asked, "Have you been hearing voices lately?"
>
> "Yes, I keep hearing 'Jesus Loves Me.' "
>
> "The song, you mean?" I asked.

132

"Yes," she answered.

Her cousin commented, "She was saved recently and has been feeling guilty for all her past sins."

"I wonder if my conversion was real," the patient stated.

Realizing the patient was a suicide risk and also that she was psychotic and inclined to hallucinate, I told the patient she should enter the hospital and I would like to see her when she got out.

This case and others we've seen in both the office and the hospital serve to illustrate typical symptoms of depression.[1-5] These symptoms have been summarized under five headings.[6] All five are not always present. The number of the five that are present depends on the severity of the depression.

Five Symptoms of Depression

Sad Affect

The depressed counselee looks depressed. His face has a dejected and discouraged appearance. His forehead is furrowed and the corners of his mouth are turned down. He either cries often or feels like it. If the depression becomes severe, the depressed individual begins to look unkempt. Men stop shaving. Women stop putting on makeup. Some depressives try to hide the depression with a smile, but the depression still shows. They have what is known as a "masked" or disguised depression.

CASE STUDY: Mrs. Z. denied feelings of depression. She was not crying and did not show many of the overt signs of depression. However, her face had the look of depression. Subsequent therapy sessions revealed that she did have masked depression.

Painful Thinking

Just as organic pain hurts physically, so does emotional pain hurt mentally. The depressive feels worthless, useless, sad, helpless, and hopeless. In fact, 75 percent of depressives feel they will never get better (they do not know that even without medication the depression will leave in about six months).[7]

Depressed patients often agonize over guilt. Not only may true guilt be present, but false guilt is also often present to a significant degree. The depressive feels guilty for all sorts of mistakes—wrongs of the past as well as those of the present. He bears a constant haunting guilt that he cannot escape. He feels responsible for events that are realistically outside his control. For some depressives, this may have as its genesis man's need to feel important.[8] The depressive feels like a nothing, like a zero. However, he cannot be a nothing, he cannot be a zero if so much hinges on him, if he is responsible for so much. Thus, as his feelings of worthlessness grow, so does the false guilt.

As the painful thinking continues, the depressive begins to withdraw. He loses his motivation. He develops a lack of interest in activities in which he was previously involved. He becomes apathetic. He begins to lose his sense of humor The future looks dim, and he eventually begins to feel that life is just not worth living. This leads to thoughts of suicide which then develop into plans and attempts at suicide. The depressive has been described as being self-possessed.[9] He is introspective and introverted. He is absorbed in melancholic and pessimistic thoughts. He feels he is inadequate or inferior in qualities that he feels are important, such as intelligence, popularity, or spiritual maturity. He may feel confused about what's really significant in his life.

CASE STUDY: Mr. Q. presented with much guilt. He felt guilty for many minor events. He would even feel guilty for failing to smile at someone and would call to apologize for it. His behavior patterns throughout life illustrate the type of individual who is prone to false guilt and depression. Such individuals are too conscientious, too concerned, too dutiful, and unable to relax. They are too serious and their conscience is too strong—it needs reeducating according to the Word of God. Such depressive counselees need to know more about God's grace, mercy, and love.

CASE STUDY: Mr. M. came to see me because he said he felt depressed. He felt blue and sad and cried often. He was sleeping poorly and had had thoughts of suicide. He was in a job that demanded much in the area of responsibility and he felt inadequate. He, too, during the course of the therapy, was able to deal with his depression, and the symptoms disappeared. When he was initially seen in therapy, he felt downhearted, blue, and sad most of the time. He said that morning was the worst part of the day. At times he cried. He had lost weight and felt tired for no reason. His heart was beating rapidly much of the time. His mind did not seem as clear as it used to, and he found it difficult to do things that he used to be able to do. He felt restless, couldn't keep still, and did not feel hopeful about the future. He was more irritable than usual and also had difficulty making decisions. Mr. M. did not feel useful and needed and felt that his life was not full. He not only did not enjoy the things he used to do but felt that others would be better off if he were dead. As stated previously, during the course of therapy, most of these symptoms did reverse themselves.

Physical Symptoms

This refers to physical changes that occur in the body with depression, the most common of which is early morning awakening. The patient awakens in the early morning hours and is not able to go back to sleep. The morning is the worst part of the day. Other forms of sleep disturbance include difficulty falling asleep or sleeping too much. In addition, there may be a disturbance in the patient's appetite so that he eats too much or too little. Thus, he may gain or lose weight. Other physiological changes occur also. For example, a tension headache, a rapid heart rate, menstrual irregularities, gastrointestinal disturbances, and diarrhea or constipation may be present. In addition, the sex drive may be lessened. Not only is the sex drive lessened, but all body activity may be decreased and slowed. His heart rate and rate of respiration may decelerate.

CASE STUDY: Mrs. D. was referred by a Christian counseling center because of severe depression. She had been markedly depressed for the last several months. She had trouble both with her sleep and her appetite and had lost about twelve pounds. She suffered from constipation. She had a rapid heartbeat at times, had low energy levels, and was tired for no apparent reason. During the course of the therapy, Mrs. D.'s somatic complaints began to clear.

Anxiety or Agitation

Anxiety often accompanies depression. The patient may not only feel the hopelessness of depression but also a great deal of tension. He may have difficulty sitting still and be more irritable than usual.

CASE STUDY: Mrs. N. asked several times as she was presenting her story to be forgiven for being so anxious and upset. She was very depressed and having much difficulty controlling her anxiety as she presented her story. She seemed irritable and even hostile. She was assured that her feelings of anxiety were understood.

Delusional Thinking (Psychosis)

Delusional thinking differs from painful thinking. In delusional thinking, the patient may imagine things that are clearly opposed to evidence, or he may hear voices. Delusions are a form of psychosis and frequently require intense treatment such as hospitalization and appropriate medications.

Widespread Occurrence of Depression

Depression is the most common symptom seen by counselors. About 8 percent of men and 16 percent of women will have a significant problem with depression during their lives.[10] It occurs twice as often in females as males.[11] It also occurs three times more often in higher socioeconomic groups.[12] About 15 percent of depressives will commit suicide.[13, 14]

A Word About Suicide

Since depression is a leading cause of suicide, a few comments about suicide are relevant. There were over 230,000 confirmed cases of suicide from 1970 to 1980, or about one every twenty minutes in the United States. Suicide is the eighth overall cause of death, and the number of attempted suicides is thought to exceed successful suicides by eight to ten times. The United States ranks at about the midpoint in suicide rates among the industrialized nations of the world.

Men commit suicide three times as often as women, but women are four times as likely to attempt suicide. Among both men and women, the highest number of completed suicides occurs after age 45. The elderly account for 25 percent of suicides, although they make up only 10 percent of the population. The suicide rate is rising most rapidly in young people, however, and for males 15 to 24 years old there was a 40 percent increase between 1970 and 1980. It is the third leading cause of death in the age group 15-to-24 years old. Divorce, unemployment, living alone, alcoholism, prior suicidal behavior, and a history of violence or rage are indicators of increased risk of suicide.[15]

A suicide attempt is usually preceded by warning signs apparent to friends, colleagues, and spouse, such as a suicide note, social isolation, giving away possessions, loss of interest in normal activities, a previous attempt and, of course, depressive symptoms such as guilt, feelings of worthlessness, and an intense wish for punishment and withdrawal. Eight of ten persons who eventually kill themselves give warnings of their intent. The risk of making a second attempt is highest within three months of the first attempt.

Only seven suicides are listed in the Scriptures. None of the men who committed suicide were in the will of God. Some of them previously had been but, of course, were not at the time of their death. The seven suicides are: Abimelech, recorded in Judges 9:54; Samson, recorded in Judges 16:30; Saul, recorded in 1 Samuel 31:4; Saul's armourbearer, recorded in 1 Samuel 31:5; Ahithophel, recorded in 2 Samuel 17:23; Zimri, recorded in 1 Kings 16:18; and Judas, recorded in the Gospels.

Causes of Depression

Authors have written about depression from centuries past to the present. They have noted it ranges from mild discouragement to psychotic proportions. Symptoms ranging from feeling a little low to those producing suicide have been noted. Causes range from physical etiologies to those produced by guilt. On the next page, are the causes or factors that we have identified as relating to the onset of depression.

Physical

Taking care of oneself with proper diet, exercise, adequate sleep, and stress reduction is essential to maintaining good mental health. Elijah, a great man of God, is a prime example of this. In the Book of 1 Kings is recorded the story of Elijah winning spiritual victories for the Lord and then plunging into discouragement. The discouragement had been preceded by his being under mental stress and probably being physically tired. Although the emotional aspects of loneliness and fear were no doubt important in the development of Elijah's discouragement, the physical factors cannot be ignored. The Lord gave Elijah food, rest, and guidance. Upon receiving these, he began to recover. Of course, Elijah had more problems than just being physically tired, but I believe this was a factor.

We, like Elijah, are prone to discouragement when we are under mental stress or are physically tired. Because of the importance of rest and nutrition, these parameters are monitored closely on a psychiatric unit. Many of one's own problems can be handled much more effectively simply by getting a good night's sleep.

Metabolic

Individuals with certain physical diseases are also more prone to depression. For example, metabolic problems such as thyroid disease and diabetes mellitus are pertinent here. For this reason, a general physical examination is in order when an individual presents with depression. With proper medication, the impact of the depression may lift.

True Guilt

Guilt may be responsible for depression. For instance, Judas felt such guilt that he committed suicide (*see* Matthew 27:5). King David also experienced much guilt and depression because of his sin with Bathsheba (*see* Psalms 32 and 51). Quoting King David, "When I kept silent *about my sin,* my body wasted away Through my groaning all day long" (Psalm 32:3 NAS). However, in contrast to Judas, David handled his guilt in a healthy manner.

Guilt may be experienced because of a sin against God or man. In the Book of Acts, for example, the Apostle Paul recorded the following, "And herein do I exercise myself, to have always a conscience void of offence toward God, and toward men" (Acts 24:16).

If the sin is against God, the solution is simple. In brief, the answer is recorded in 1 John 1:9. Quoting the Apostle John, "If we confess [agree with God about] our sins, he is faithful and just to forgive us our sins, and to cleanse us from all unrighteousness." Once an individual asks God to forgive him for a sin, God forgives and remembers the sin no more. The individual may still feel guilty if he has not thoroughly learned of the mercy of God, but this guilt is not of God.

Although all sins are against God, some also affect people, and although God completely forgives the sin, an obligation exists toward a person offended. The love of Christ constrains us to ask forgiveness of those we have offended. However, I do not believe one should search in the past for possible sins and individuals he has offended, but rather that if the Holy Spirit continues to convict of a particular offense, the issue should be settled. The apology should not contain unnecessary and embarrassing details, and it should be only to the one offended. Finally, in apologizing when one is only partially at fault, he will be more effective if he uses wording that places the responsibility upon himself rather than both himself and the other person. Otherwise the other individual will become defensive, and the purpose of the apology will be defeated.

False Guilt

Christians with obsessive-compulsive personalities will be prone to depression. An obsessive-compulsive personality type has been well documented by observation to be a specific personality pattern. This personality is characterized by being overly rigid, conscientious, and perfectionistic. Moreover, this type of person is absorbed in right and wrong, and, being overly dutiful, he is unable to relax or have fun. To be sure, his conscience is stricter than God Himself. Whereas in sociopaths, the conscience is underdeveloped, in obsessive-compulsive individuals, the conscience is overdeveloped. In either case, the issue is not so much what the individual thinks, but what the Word of God says. An obsessive-compulsive individual needs to educate himself repeatedly concerning the grace and mercy of God. Rather than being absorbed in the letter of the law, he would benefit from the thought expressed by Christ in the following words, ". . . the words that I speak unto you, they are spirit, and they are life" (John 6:63). He needs to relax and enjoy part of the abundant life that God desires for him (*see* John 10:10). And concerning his numerous worries, the advice of Apostle Paul is applicable:

> Finally, brethren, whatsoever things are true, whatsoever things are honest, whatsoever things are just, whatsoever things are pure, whatsoever things are lovely, whatsoever things are of good report; if there be any virtue, and if there be any praise, think on these things.
>
> PHILIPPIANS 4:8

Misplaced Guilt

Whether true, false, or misplaced, it is feasible that any emotionally drained individual may feel guilty for some sin in the past and displace guilt to numerous insignificant areas.

Anger Turned Inward

Depression has been defined as anger turned inward. This anger may be the result of the loss of a love object. This love object varies from a loved one to self-esteem. If the loved object is another person, the patient becomes very angry with the individual, then turns the anger toward himself, and thus becomes depressed. The anger may also be the result of the violation of one's "rights."[16]

In either case, bitterness and then depression result. Thus, if a Christian is wronged, what should he do? If he holds his anger in and becomes bitter, he runs the risk of depression. Anger can often be expressed in an appropriate way verbally, and a better and closer relationship develops between persons. Often a person needs to be more assertive. This is especially true in depressed people. Yet, he does not believe in letting his anger show at the expense of hurting others unnecessarily. The following are helpful steps for dealing with anger:

- Realize that there may be bitterness toward another or others.
- List those who have offended.
- Forgive them because of the love of Christ (*see* Matthew 6:12) and because depression is too high a price to pay.
- Give up "rights" (*see* Philippians 3:7). Since depression may be anger turned inward and since anger usually results from a violation of what one considers to be his rights, one solution for bitterness is to give up one's "rights" to God. The question that may be asked is, "Who is smarter, God or I?"

Christians often consider time, their cars, their health, and the like to be "rights." However, God desires to give these back to us as privileges. If one has no rights, they cannot be violated, and one cannot thus become angry. Of course, because of the tendency to reclaim privileges as rights, this yielding is not a one-time occasion.

- Talk it out. One should not express anger at the expense of hurting others unnecessarily. However, others often need things pointed out to them. Sitting down and talking with another in an appropriate manner (*see* Galatians 6:1) can be very helpful for both and helps to externalize rather than internalize the anger.
- Express emotionally charged energy in exercise. This gives one the opportunity to express and release pent-up energy. It also allows time to become more objective.

Self-Effort

A major reason for discouragement among dedicated Christians is their trying to live and work for Christ in their own strength. Clearly, the Christian life is a supernatural life and can only be lived through the power of the Holy Spirit. Thus,

Apostle Paul stated, "I can do all things through Christ . . ." (Philippians 4:13) and again he stated, ". . . it is God which worketh in you both to will and to do of his good pleasure" (Philippians 2:13). In contrast, in Romans 7:24, he recorded his discouragement that resulted from trying to live for God in his own energy.

If the Lord has a ministry He wants accomplished and if an individual is available, God will accomplish what He desires. To be sure, wrong priorities and assuming responsibilities (even in Christian activities) beyond what God desires is a major cause of discouragement. God is mostly concerned with an individual's really getting to know Him (*see* Philippians 3:10 AMPLIFIED); second, with his meeting the needs of his family (*see* 1 Timothy 5:8); and third, with ministering to others in the particular ways God has chosen for him. Often this endless self-effort is the result of fear of rejection by God.

Wrong Perspective

Psalm 73 tells of the discouragement and depression that came to King David as a result of a wrong perspective.[17]

"But as for me, my feet were almost gone; my steps had well nigh slipped. For I was envious at the foolish, when I saw the prosperity of the wicked" (Psalm 73:2, 3).

Likewise, many things that God has not chosen to give an individual today may appear very inviting to him. He may forget the only two tangible things that are going to last—the Word of God and people (*see* Matthew 24:35 and 1 John 4:11, 12). These are the things that are really important. He may temporarily forget that the inner love, joy, and peace he wants are the results of the fruit of the Spirit (*see* Galatians 5:22, 23) and not material or worldly things.

In verses 16 and 17 of Psalm 73, King David recorded the moment when his perspective changed. He stated, "When I thought to know this, it was too painful for me; Until I went into the sanctuary of God; then understood I their end." This sanctuary for each Christian today may be different. It may be getting away to relax. It may be memorizing some particular verses.

It may be having more fellowship with Christians. It may be getting out and sharing Christ with others.

King Solomon's conclusion after seeking fulfillment in life from humanitarianism, sex, amusement, education, and pleasure was ". . . vanity of vanities; all is vanity" (Ecclesiastes 1:2). That statement sounds like an answer from a modern-day, depressed patient. Solomon's record of his search for fulfillment is found in two books in the Bible that are back to back.[18] One is Ecclesiastes, in which Solomon records his search by means described in sources above. The second book is Song of Solomon. This book is an analogy of a human love relationship to Christ and His Church. If we carry the logic, the analogy represents the relationship found in a well-balanced life of Bible study, prayer, fellowship, and witnessing. This perspective is found only through an intimate, cultivated fellowship with Christ Himself and healthy relationships with fellow Christians.

Adjustment Reactions

I have often used the diagnosis of *adjustment reaction* in psychiatry to describe a particularly stressful time in life for any given individual.

One major category of depression has been called *exogenous depression,* which means that the depression comes from without rather than within the individual. The individual is reacting to external stress. There is nothing abnormal about feeling acutely stressed or down at times, although it is detrimental to remain that way. There is nothing wrong with being perplexed (*see* 2 Corinthians 4:8, 9), but it is wrong to carry this to despair. Being perplexed drives us to Christ, but remaining in despair results in depression.

Attacks by Satan

When one feels discouraged or uncomfortable, how can he be sure God is not trying to tell him something? While attending a Navigators' Christian conference, I was exposed to the following points that are helpful:[19]

	GOD	*SATAN or Possibly SELF*
a.	The individual can identify a specific problem accounting for his discouragement. However, caution should be used because this is not necessarily from God.	The reason for discouragement may remain vague. Confusion is a prominent feature, and God is not the author of confusion (*see* 1 Corinthians 14:33).
b.	The individual senses there is hope.	The individual feels hopeless.
c.	The person senses he can be built up through dealing with his problems.	The person feels downgraded.

A Learned Response

Although there is no current diagnosis of depressive personality, it seems there are many people who are just habitually depressed. In some families, the children are indirectly taught that the appropriate way to handle stress is to become depressed. Depression is acceptable in these families. Several members in the family may suffer from depression. Depression becomes a learned response. These individuals go through life depressed, and depression seems to have become a part of their personalities. In these individuals depression may become a powerful tool by which to manipulate others. Thus, a young child may learn to get attention when he is depressed, and the learned response is reinforced.

Endogenous Depression

One way depression has been categorized is by describing it as *endogenous* or *exogenous*. As stated previously, the exogenous depression is caused by a person's reaction to external stress. On the other hand, endogenous depression comes totally from within the individual. Exogenous depression has been a favorite subject of psychiatric articles through the years.[20]

The foundation for exogenous depression could start very early in life. During the interview, the counselor often notes a history of a cold, rejecting mother. The baby felt rejected. In fact, he started to expect everyone to reject him just as his mother did. This expectation of rejection led to feelings of hostility. To avoid getting close to others and thus avoid being rejected, the patient started projecting his hostile feelings onto others and imagining they did not want to get to know him. He is hostile toward others but imagines they are hostile toward him. He does not want to become close to others but imagines they do not want to be close to him. The avoidance of being close to anyone left the patient with a host of unmet dependency needs. To compensate for these needs, the depressive may become superindependent. He may become a superman-independent, a friend to all who need help.

If we examine the above, we can see that a cycle has been set up. The cycle alternates between feelings of rejection, unmet dependency needs, hostility, projection of the hostility, and avoidance of close relationships. The following story has been told to illustrate the cycle.

> A depressive is driving down a country road and has a flat tire. He looks in his trunk for a jack. Not finding one, he spots a farmhouse one-quarter mile away with a truck in the front yard and says to himself, "I'll go borrow his jack." As he approaches the house he is feeling bad (1) for failing to have a jack, and (2) for having to depend on someone else for help. As he gets nearer the farmhouse, he begins to expect rejection and to get angry over what is his expectation of rejection. He becomes more and more angry at unmet dependency needs (projects the anger he feels toward himself for needing the jack), so that by the time he knocks on the door, the farmer opens the door and the depressive yells, "Keep your jack." This will usually guarantee that he doesn't get the jack and he walks back reconvinced that you can't depend on people.[21]

The patient can really benefit from insights into these behavior patterns. He can learn that *he can change rejection* by others by changing his rejections of them. He can learn he does have dependency needs and how to *meet those dependency needs* in appropriate ways. He can begin to learn that no one can be a superman, and *no one is perfect.* He can begin to *recognize his feelings* and to deal with them and his anger more appropriately. He can recognize that although these behavior patterns may have started in early life, *he can change them.*

Other Causes

There are several other causes of depression. For example, postpartum depression is a particular subset of depression. This depression following the birth of a child is not uncommon. Another depression that seems to have unique features is the depression seen during adolescence. This depression is especially different in that the symptoms are often different from the symptoms seen in adults. Rather than having a sad facial expression and crying often, the adolescent starts to "act out" socially. He may steal, lie, or "act out" sexually.

Mention should also be made of problems that simulate depression but are not depression itself. For example, grief is not depression. It is grief and is very normal. Also, certain personality types, such as hysterics, will present with the chief complaint of depression. Further evaluation may reveal this to be more a presenting complaint rather than the real problem.

Nine Ways of Dealing with Depression

Medication

Antidepressive medication doses produce significant improvement in mood, sleep, and appetite, and thus the individual is better able to deal with his problems. In depression there may be an actual chemical abnormality, and antidepressive medication corrects this abnormality. In addition, it works in other ways to improve mood, sleep, and appetite.

For example, antidepressants (*tricyclics*) have effects on the following systems:[22]

- Limbic structures. The effect here results in improved mood.

- Hypothalamus. The effect here results in improved appetite and other biologic functions.
- Reticular activating system (inhibited). The effect here results in improved sleep.
- Neurohumoral deposits. These are increased with medication, and this may account for much of the beneficial effects.

Some Christian counselors have, in the past, been opposed to medications that affect the brain's function. We believe that an understanding of how the medication works in the correction of a chemical imbalance is important in considering the validity of that medication. If the medication works to correct an actual biochemical abnormality and returns the body back to its usual physiologic state, we believe the use is valid. For example, who would argue with the use of insulin to return a diabetic to a normal physiologic state? In like manner, some drugs used in psychiatry serve simply to return the body back to a balanced physiologic state. For example, the antidepressive medications (tricyclics) build norepinephrine, a neurotransmitter in the brain which is important in returning the emotional state back to a normal level. The tricyclics (antidepressants) serve to block the re-uptake of norepinephrine at the nerve endings, thereby increasing the norepinephrine in the synapse between the nerve cells. When this level becomes normal, much of the depression disappears. Of course, the basic problems must still be dealt with in order to really help the patient. The medications serve to help the patient become mentally functional through balancing the biochemistry of the brain so the patient can then progress in therapy.

On the other hand, if the medications do not correct an abnormal physiologic state, we would question their validity. For example, the "recreational" use of amphetamines may give an artificial lift to mood. However, they do not restore the body to a balanced physiologic state, and in a couple of weeks, the depression returns stronger than ever.

A Friend

A warm and understanding friend who will listen is of great help to a depressed person. Often the depressed patient has low self-esteem. In this case, a friend can help the individual to have a healthy estimate of himself (*see* Romans 12:3). This is done not by simply telling him that he is important (although healthy words that uplift are crucial) but also by proving it to him by actions that show interest in him.

A Focus on Behavior

If there is no apparent cause for the depression, the depressed person should focus on daily planned activities, avoiding those activities that would tend to produce more depression, and practicing activities that are priority. For example, the following are practical suggestions:

- Avoid soap operas
- Get up early
- Go to work regardless of feelings
- Have sufficient times with family
- Do something nice for your mate
- Have time of enjoyment with others

In other words, focus on behavior, not just feelings. It is important to let the counselee ventilate and talk out his feelings; this helps to deal with the internalized anger that has caused the depression and helps to bring the anxiety from the subconscious (where it cannot be dealt with appropriately) to the conscious. This also helps the counselee to feel the counselor cares for him and understands him. However, the counselor must move beyond just dealing with feelings and also deal with behavior. Indeed, we have little direct control over our feelings, but maximum control over our behavior.[23] The patient will benefit by developing new interests and activities. The Bible acknowledges that feelings are important (*see* Hebrews 4:15) but it also puts a great emphasis on the importance of behavior.[24] (*See* Philippians 4:13; 2:13; James 1:22; Genesis 4:6, 7).

Prayer

Verbally expressing troubles in prayer is helpful. King David said that morning, noon, and night he would pray and cry *aloud*. Just ventilating alone would help, but how much more helpful it is to share with God who has the power to give a ". . . sound mind" (*see* 2 Timothy 1:7).

Bible

The Word of God gives joy to counteract depression. Thus Jeremiah said, "Thy words were found, and I did eat them; and thy word was unto me the joy and rejoicing of mine heart: for I am called by thy name, O Lord God of hosts" (Jeremiah 15:16). To be sure, the Word of God is ". . . quick, and powerful . . ." (Hebrews 4:12).

Fellowship

If one is around other Christians with joy, he will catch it. Solomon stated, "Iron sharpeneth iron; so a man sharpeneth the countenance of his friend" (Proverbs 27:17).

Focus on a Plan

In particularly stressful situations that are producing discouragement, formulate a plan of action.[25] List all alternatives of what to do, and then try the one chosen.

Focus on Assertiveness

The depressed patient is often very unassertive. In fact, he can hardly say *no* to anyone when asked to do something. If the patient can become healthily assertive, he will probably improve. It is helpful to encourage the patient to say *no* when what he is requested to do is not on his priority list (God, family, joy, ministry) and is not really helpful to the other person. Likewise, if the patient can appropriately express his feelings, he will probably improve. Rather than being too assertive, the depressed person has often gone to the other extreme and does not speak up when he should.

Insight

Insight is very important. It involves looking for the situation and facing it without distortion, as it really is, no matter how painful or repulsive. Insight is also the understanding and acceptance of when the depression began and what maintains the depression. Insight is also the taking in and willingness to apply those steps necessary to change the patterns of behavior and depression.

Favour is deceitful, and beauty is
vain: but a woman that feareth the
Lord, she shall be praised.
PROVERBS 31:30

8 The Hysterical Woman and the Sociopathic Man

A Psychiatric Survey

Dr. Minirth shares the following observation:

During my residency in psychiatry, I did a categorical survey of the types of patients I had during a six-month rotation on the psychiatric ward. These findings were obtained:

- 30%—Hysterical trends, personality or neurosis
- 20%—Depression/anxiety
- 10%—Drug-related problems
- 15%—Psychotic

The patients also revealed the following:

- 60%—females (40% males)
- The most frequent age was 20 to 35 years. The number of teenagers and individuals over fifty was also significant.
- The overwhelming majority of patients indicated they wanted help very much.
- Most had some type of religious training, and a significant number were Christians.

Conclusions are difficult to draw from such a small sample of a patient population (approximately 40), but one can conclude with certainty that individuals with emotional conflicts are in

151

search of help. One may also conclude that being a Christian does not necessarily free one of emotional turmoil.

In my particular survey, I found *hysteria* was the most common problem. This certainly does not document that this is the main emotional problem today. However, judging from other observations, it does seem to be a prevalent problem if we use the term in a broad sense. Solomon probably dealt with the sensuous (hysterical and seductive) woman more than any other single issue, which again documents the importance and magnitude of the problem.

One characteristic of an hysterical personality is that of being seductive. However, it should be pointed out that although the hysterical personality is often seductive, the reverse is not always true. All sensuous women are not hysterical.

Our society is increasingly focusing on the sensuous woman. Thus, many advertisements are based on sexual appeals, as are many movies. The irony of the situation is that, although the sensuous (hysterical and seductive) woman is presented as outwardly inviting and warm, she is inwardly lonely and frustrated. Hence, she appears as a great sex partner, but in reality she often never reaches a climax or orgasm. She may appear as loving, but inside she feels bitterness, which prevents a warm, loving relationship with free sexual expression. She desires love and affection, and thus by seductive dress and actions she attempts to obtain these, but the close interaction she seeks is blocked by her subconscious fears.

If Christian women have these tendencies and do not find God's answers, they will live frustrated lives. Likewise, if Christian men marry women with these traits, they, too, will live disappointed lives unless they know how to deal with their problems and values.

Psychiatric Examples

The following summarizes common features in patients with hysterical trends:

1. Mrs. S. complained that she was depressed. She had been treated by a couple of psychiatrists in the past for depression, but it was becoming worse.

Comment: These women may seem depressed, and sympathetic counselors may be manipulated by this However, depression is only the surface and not the root problem. Recognizing this in this particular lady and applying some other principles, Dɪ Minirth was able to help her These principles are shared later

2. Mrs. J. presented to the psychiatric unit because of a suɪcidal gesture.

Comment: There is often a history of several rather feeble suicide gestures. These are usually manipulative in nature. In fact, although men are three times as apt to die by suicide, women attempt suicide four times more.

3. Mrs. T. had been married several times and her present marriage was unstable.

Comment: These women seem to repeatedly find an idealized male, marry him, become disappointed, and then divorce him.

To account for this, the psychoanalytic school has proposed the following theory: The idealized male represents the patient's father. Disappointment comes because the male turns out not to be perfect, just like the father. Ambivalence for men is reinforced. Hence, unresolved conflicts between father and daughter still cause problems. Disappointment comes because of deepseated bitterness the patient has toward her father and, thus, toward men in general.

4. Mrs. A. was seductive in her dress and actions.

Comment: This partially results because the woman wants to be accepted and loved, as commented before. One possible reason for her being seductive is having learned as a young child that she could gain attention from her father by such behavior. This pattern was continued in relationships with other men.

5. Mrs. M. tended to be dramatic, vain, excitable, emotionally unstable, and immature. At one time in her life, she had been close to the Lord and had been happy. During one interview Dr. Minirth shared the following:

> "You apparently have a real need for someone to care for you, and there is someone who wants to know you more than you want to know Him."

"Who?" she asked
"Christ," I answered
She agreed and we proceeded to outline her responsibilities
and a plan that could aid in reestablishing a true inward peace

It should be pointed out that men may also have hysterical personalities Possibly men are diagnosed less often for this for several reasons First, Greeks set the trend of diagnosing only
women with this problem when they said it was due to a migrating
uterus and, therefore, applied only to women. Second, men are
usually the ones who make the diagnosis, and they may be biased
in their conclusions. Third, a male with these characteristics (manipulative, self-centered, feeling little guilt, etc.) might be commonly diagnosed as *sociopathic* rather than *hysterical*

Treatment of Hysteria

Therapy is dealt with in later chapters, but briefly, there are
generally three points we use in therapy with a hysteric.

First, one must consider the need for medication. Of course,
there is no medication for immaturity. However, hysterics can
become very depressed or anxious. Some depression and anxiety can be helpful because it motivates a person to change.
However, if the depression is extreme, one runs the risk of
suicide, and antidepressive medication should be considered.

Second, the counselor must consider what type of approach
and attitude he will use. In general, the counselor wants to be
warm and friendly. However, since hysterics may misinterpret
this and since they are very manipulative, an adult-to-adult or
matter-of-fact approach proves best.

Third, in counseling sessions the counselor should use a
reality-oriented type of approach. The patient needs to look at
her behavior in reality. For example, does she realize she is
being seductive? What is she willing to do about it? This patient
concentrates on feelings and neglects logic. She needs to be
encouraged to think about what she is doing, to think logically
and rationally, and to think more and feel less. We have found
it helpful to confront the patient with her irresponsible behavior

and then help her plan appropriate behavior and methods to deal with specific problems.

It is very interesting to compare current psychiatric views of the hysterical personality with those of the Bible concerning the seductive woman. This illustrates that the Bible is as modern and relevant today as it was in the early Church. We should mention that in the following descriptions only a general comparison can be made. The psychiatric description is only of the personality type having prominent hysterical characteristic traits.

The Hysterical Woman
The Bible and Psychiatry Compared

Psychiatry	Bible
1. She is manipulative.	1. She ". . . flatters with her words . . ." (Proverbs 2:16 NAS). " . . smoother than oil is her speech . " (Proverbs 5:3 NAS).
2. She may be characterized by a series of marriages and divorces.	2. She ". . . leaves the companion of her youth . . ." (Proverbs 2:17 NAS).
3. She does not think. When working with this type of personality, psychiatrists are taught to help the patient to think because she goes through life feeling much but really thinking little.	3. She does not ponder the path of life . " (Proverbs 5:6 NAS).
4. She is emotionally unstable.	4. ". . . her ways are unstable . . ." (Proverbs 5:6 NAS).
5. She is vain and self-centered.	5. She is outwardly beautiful but inwardly vain and self-centered (Proverbs 6:25; 7:10–21 NAS).

Psychiatry	Bible
6. She may be seductive in her mannerisms.	6. She is seductive in both dress and actions (*see* Proverbs 7:10–21 NAS). "... she seduces him" (Proverbs 7:21 NAS). "... catch you with her eyelids" (Proverbs 6:25 NAS). "... dressed as a harlot ..." (Proverbs 7:10 NAS).
7. She is dependent on others. She uses the defense of rationalization.	7. She rationalizes in her mind for her impurity. She feels no guilt (*see* Proverbs 30:20 NAS).
8. Her basic motivation is hatred. Psychoanalysis in effect teaches that the basic motivation behind the hysterical woman is hatred for men.	8. She desires the downfall of her lover. "... many are the victims she has cast down ..." (Proverbs 7:26 NAS).
9. She is overreactive and dramatic.	9. "She is boisterous and rebellious ..." (Proverbs 7:11 NAS).
10. She is naive. Although outwardly seductive and a woman of the world, she is basically very naive and really is often sexually frigid.	10. "She is naive ... (Proverbs 9:13 NAS).
11. She is attention seeking.	11. She is attention seeking (*see* Proverbs 7:10–21 NAS).
12. Prognosis poor without intervention.	12. Prognosis is poor (*see* Proverbs 2:18). But there is reason to be optimistic, and there is hope (*see* account of Jesus and the woman of Sychar in John 4).

The Sociopathic Man

The counterpart of the hysterical woman is the sociopathic man. It would seem that, if psychiatrists see certain traits in a woman, they tend to diagnose her as hysterical, whereas if they see similar traits in a man, they tend to diagnose him as sociopathic. As in a hysterical personality, the sociopathic personality is characterized by being self-centered and immature. He is out for himself and, in fact, seldom forms close personal relations with anyone.

In the survey listed at the beginning of this chapter, Dr. Minirth noted that 10 percent of those patients had an alcohol or drug-related problem. A significant percent of them had sociopathic traits. And this is in keeping with *sociopathy*, for often sociopaths do have an alcohol- or drug-related problem. As stated earlier, these individuals are characterized by a lack of conscience. They do not feel guilt for wrongdoings. They do not seem to learn from experience. Yet, they are charming and likable, having traits that facilitate an ability to manipulate people. They feel they are okay and the rest of the world is not okay.

PSYCHIATRY	BIBLE: ROMANS 1
1. Repeated conflict with society	Murder, deceit, disobedient to parents
2. Incapable of loyalty to others	Full of envy, spiteful, covenant breakers, backbiters
3. Selfish	Covetous, full of envy, proud boasters
4. Callous	Filled with unrighteousness
5. Not able to learn from experience	Without understanding

Treatment of the Sociopathic Man

First, a comment about medicine would be helpful. A sociopath, as anyone else, can become anxious or depressed; but the therapist would be especially careful about giving this individual any medicine because of his tendency to abuse drugs. In fact, he often comes into therapy with the ulterior motive of obtaining drugs.

Second, the counselor must again consider what type of attitude will work best. Usually, a matter-of-fact or confrontational approach works best.

Third, the counselor must consider whether he is willing to work with this individual. We have heard psychiatrists cynically commenting on the undependability of sociopaths, "Diagnose them and then discharge them."

As Christians, we have more hope. Sociopaths can become Christians. They can understand the Gospel and put their faith in Christ. We believe this is their main hope. We should also mention that many of them will improve with age, for they seem to "burn out," or expend the energy they devote to themselves.

Interestingly, one of the most useful areas for applying observations about the counselee's personality type is in the area of marriage counseling. Numerous combinations could be formed. However, several of the combinations seem to occur more often and have been described in detail.[1] Of course, most marriages will not be as sick as the ones listed below. However, many of the traits may be present in a less severe form.

Types of Marital Combinations

One of the most common types of marriages in America is the obsessive-compulsive man and the hysterical woman. The obsessive-compulsive man is dutiful, conscientious, and concerned and has a strict conscience. He is attracted to a female who is somewhat the opposite of him in many ways—a woman who is emotional, excitable, dramatic, theatrical, and seductive. He finds this dramatic, emotional, seductive nature pleasant at first. She arouses pleasurable emotions in him.

Likewise, she is attracted to him since he has many opposite traits than she. She likes his nonemotional, stable, logical, father-figure image.

Each finds in the other what he lacks. He lacks emotions. She arouses this in him. She lacks logic and stability. She likes the apparent stability she finds in him. Thus, while they can really complement (since he can't feel and she can't think), they may begin to become irritated with each other. He may grow tired of her dramatics, and she may grow tired of his cold logic. If both are relatively immature, the stage is set for a lifelong battle of conflicting personality traits.

A second type of marriage is the passive-aggressive husband married to the passive-aggressive wife. Both are passive and immature. Both want to receive more than they give. Both are overly dependent. Neither is able to understand the needs of the other because they are so self-centered.

Dr. Minirth had one such couple in marriage counseling. Both claimed the other was immature, self-centered, childish, and just wanted his own way. They seemed surprised when their psychological test showed they were extremely similar in personality type. Indeed, both were immature and self-centered. Each had been able to recognize it in the other but had been blinded to their own personal problems.

A third type of marriage that is often seen in America and is based on a neurotic attraction is the passive husband and the dominant wife. Each feels a neurotic need of the other. He has a need for someone to lead, to be in charge, and to dominate. She has a need to lead, to control, and to dominate. Conflicts arise because he is inwardly hostile at being dominated, and she is frustrated by not having her own dependency needs met. This, too, is a parent-child type interaction, but here she is the parent and he is the child.

A fourth type of marriage is that of the paranoid husband and the depressive wife. That is the sadomasochistic type relationship. He is jealous, hostile, angry, and has a need to hurt others. She is prone to depression, has a low self-image, and readily accepts blame. In short, she has a need to be hurt. His main defense mechanism is *projection,* by which he attributes his own shortcomings to her. Her main defense mechanism is *introjection,* by which she assumes blame for things she didn't do. Often, the female in this relationship had critical, demanding parents. She subconsciously sought out the same type of parental figure in the man she married. Accepting blame became a way of life.

A fifth type of marriage is the paranoid wife and the depressive husband. It is just the opposite of number four above. In this relationship the wife is angry, hostile, and paranoid. The man has a low self-image and readily accepts blame. The same sadomasochistic neurotic needs exist as above. She has the need to hurt others, and he has a need to be hurt. In a warped sort of way, accepting blame gives the depressive husband a little self-worth. He feels like he is nothing, but he can't be a nothing if he is responsible for so much.

A sixth type of relationship is the asthenic wife and the obsessive-compulsive husband. She is sick (both mentally and physically) and has a need for someone to totally take care of her. He feels inadequate in the world and has a need to take care of someone who is weaker than he is. Conflicts arise because she begins to resent being totally dependent on someone else, and he begins to resent the drain he feels from her continuing sickness.

A seventh type of marital relationship is that of the obsessive-compulsive husband and the obsessive-compulsive wife. Both may be overly perfectionistic, demanding, and critical. Thus, they can hardly live with themselves and certainly have difficulty with each other. Of course, if they are relatively healthy with their obsessive-compulsiveness, they can have a very orderly marriage.

The technique of counseling will be dealt with in a later chapter. Let it suffice here to say that the marriage counselor has various roles. He is a listener. He is an observer of communication patterns. He is one who confronts and points out games and detrimental defense mechanisms. He helps the couple gain insight into their personality types. He helps them to formulate specific plans of action for dealing with their problems.

Part III

Treating Emotional Problems

To every thing there is a season, and
a time to every purpose under the
heaven . . . a time to keep silence,
and a time to speak.

ECCLESIASTES 3:1, 7

9   Indirect-Directive Counseling

Principles in Counseling

Christian counseling is many-faceted, but basically there are
three aspects that must be present for counseling to be effective.
The first aspect has to do with the counselor's relationship to
Jesus Christ. As in any work for God, we are only the instru-
ments through which God works, and the real effectiveness of
the work depends on God. The second aspect has to do with
certain attributes the counselor needs to become involved in a
meaningful way with the patient. It involves really caring for the
patient. This is what patients want to find. Caring is something
patients can sense, and the relationship that develops because of
this is of paramount importance in helping the patient. Thus,
more important than the type of counseling used is the personality of the counselor. The third aspect has to do with the type
of counseling approach used. We have found that generally an
indirect-directive type of approach has been the most effective.
This is the topic of this chapter. The other two aspects will be
discussed later.

Directive Versus Non-Directive Counseling

Counseling breaks down into two broad divisions: *directive*
and *non-directive*. The therapies of William Glasser and Carl
Rogers illustrate this. Glasser would be considered directive and

Rogers indirective. Without a doubt, men through the years have lost balance in extremes in one direction or the other Psychiatrists in the past have been criticized for being non-directive, and we would agree. Yet we have concerns that some Christian counselors have erred in being too directive rather than helping an individual form a value judgment for himself.

If a counselor is too non-directive, he is not fair to the counselee. Counselees consult others whom they feel have wisdom and can guide them in an appropriate direction. The counselor owes the patient this.

If a counselor is too directive, however, he defeats his own purpose. A decision will last only if it is a personal conviction. The following example illustrates the point:

Dr. Minirth relates a case in which one Christian friend was telling another Christian friend that he was definitely living in the wrong location and that he should move to an area where God wanted him to be. The counselor giving the advice was very dogmatic, perhaps made his friend defensive, and apparently did not succeed in helping him develop his own value judgment. While the counselor giving the advice may have been very correct in his thinking, his method proved ineffective.

We do not wish to discredit the importance of being direct when indicated. In fact, Christ was often very direct, as were Elihu, Solomon, and Apostle Paul. Christ was directive at times and non-directive at other times. In Matthew 13 is recorded an instance when He taught the people in parables and thus was less than overtly directive (*see* Matthew 13:3). However, in Matthew 19 is recorded an instance when He was very directive with a rich young man (*see* Matthew 19:21–23). The point is that each individual must be dealt with as an individual, and the approach must be tailored. For example, hysterics respond frequently to a more directive approach to counseling, but obsessive-compulsive patients often respond best to non-directive techniques. In either case, the value judgment can only be made by the counselee.

It should be noted that we use the term "indirect" rather than "non-direct" in describing our counseling style. Technically, they are not the same, and we are referring to direct and indirect counseling rather than direct and non-direct counseling. However, we doubt that any therapist is ever truly non-directive, for we are directive with every move we make

The approach is directive in that the counselor should know what the counselee needs to do to handle his problems and how to guide him in that direction. The counselor should be able to recognize the problem and approach it accordingly Also, because the Bible is the Christian counselor's standard of authority, his counseling is directive His goals are to help the counselee solve his problems in accordance with the Will of God and to help the counselee grow spiritually. Inasmuch as the Bible is the counselor's foundation and guide, his counseling is directive.

The approach is indirect in that the counselor often uses indirect techniques (questions, suggestive statements, listening) to help the counselee reach appropriate decisions. The counselor uses *indirect* techniques for a *directed* end. If a decision is a counselee's own, it will be much more meaningful and lasting.

In 2 Samuel, Nathan, a prophet of God, used this method. King David had sinned with the wife of Uriah the Hittite. This displeased the Lord, and He sent Nathan to rebuke David. Nathan was very intelligent, and he knew the dangers of rebuking a king. Thus, he had to help the king obtain valuable insight without giving direct advice. He must have known that we often react to the shortcomings in others because they are present in ourselves. So, he proceeded to tell King David the following story and accomplished his objective. The verses that follow may be thought of as King David on Trial.

> Then the Lord sent Nathan to David. And he came to him, and said, "There were two men in one city, the one rich and the other poor. The rich man had a great many flocks and herds. But the poor man had nothing except one little ewe lamb Which he bought and nourished; and it grew up together with him and his children. It would eat of his bread and drink of his cup and lie in his bosom, And was like a daughter to him. Now a traveler came to the rich man, And he was unwilling to take from his own flock or his own herd, To prepare for the wayfarer who had come to him; Rather he

took the poor man's ewe lamb and prepared it for the one who had
come to him."

Then David's anger burned greatly against the man, and he said
to Nathan, "As the Lord lives, surely the man who has done this
deserves to die. And he must make restitution for the lamb four-
fold, because he did this thing and had no compassion."

Nathan then said to David, "You are the man! . . ."
2 SAMUEL 12:1–7 NAS

Christ—The Approach He Used in Counseling

Christ was a master at helping others obtain valuable insights.
He did this through statements, questions, and parables. His
statements were at times stern and rebuking, but at other times
they were kind and gentle. Likewise, the types of questions He
asked varied. The Gospel according to Mark records approximately twenty questions that were asked by Christ. Nearly half
of the twenty questions were directed at either the Pharisees,
the religious leaders of the day, or the multitudes. A couple of
questions were directed at individuals. Most of the questions
seemed matter-of-fact, and their purpose was most often to teach
or help others gain insight. And while Christ was kind and loving, He remained objective, and at least five of the twenty questions (three directed at the Pharisees and two directed at the
disciples) were rebuking and cutting in nature.

The Counseling Process

Effective counseling frequently involves the art of asking questions. Questions force others to think and reach their own conclusions when declarations might be disregarded. The ability to
help others gain insights by questions is largely learned and, in
trained hands, is one of the most valuable tools a counselor has.

The Present Versus the Past—Feelings Versus Behavior

One pendulum in counseling seems to be swinging from focusing on the past to focusing on the "here and now." Another
pendulum also seems to be swinging from focusing on feelings to
focusing on behavior.

There are two extremes when considering the importance of the past. One is to blame the past for present, inappropriate behavior. This extreme in counseling focuses almost entirely on the past. The other extreme tends to avoid the past entirely, and counseling centers around the present only. We have found that a balanced view works best. In counseling, we focus mostly on present behavior and specific plans to deal with problems while realizing that unresolved issues that occurred in the past must be dealt with appropriately. It must be recognized that the past forms much of an individual's personality, and although an individual is responsible for present behavior, early environmental stresses can cause an individual to be more prone to detrimental defense mechanisms. The first five years of life are a major factor in determining whether an individual will be an extrovert, introvert, leader, follower, quiet, loud, dramatic, or shy. Thus, in agreement with reality therapy, we focus on the present but will deal with or listen to the past as indicated.

There are also the extremes of feelings and behavior. One school will focus entirely on feelings in counseling, the other will refuse to allow the counselee to talk about feelings at all. The Bible recognizes the importance of feelings (*see* Hebrews 4:15), but it places much emphasis on behavior. We should understand our feelings but not let them rule us. The founders of reality therapy have well expressed the importance of behavior in their statement that one has maximum control over his behavior but minimum control over his feelings.

In summary, we would offer the following three suggestions to Christian counselors to help them offer balanced and effective care for their counselees:

Genuinely care. Caring is something that is intangible but that people can really sense. This is especially true in individuals with problems. We all gravitate to people who are warm, understanding, accepting, personal, and who will listen to us. These qualities are of utmost importance for the Christian counselor (*see* Galatians 4:19; Romans 1:11, 12; John 17:19–21).

Caring results in the building of a relationship. The relationship that exists determines much of the progress of therapy.

Without a relationship, a commitment from a counselee means little. Without a relationship, the counselee is often not motivated to change.

Use an indirect-directive approach. This may sound like a play on words, but we have found this approach to be the key foundation of counseling. Again, by the term "indirect-directive," we mean that the approach is directive in the sense that the counselor knows what direction would be healthy for the one counseled and guides him in that direction. It is also directive because God's Word is the counselor's standard of authority. The approach is indirect in its *guidance* because, unless a person reaches his own decisions, he is not likely to benefit. Christ often used questions to help others reach decisions. As was mentioned earlier, approximately twenty questions are recorded that Christ asked. Open-ended questions, leading questions, and teaching questions have all been of great help. If a young person is told, for example, that only two things will last (God's Word and people), he might remember this for a short period. On the contrary, if he is asked what two things will last and he comes up with the solution, this will more likely remain in his memory. Without a doubt, counselors through the years have lost balance by becoming either too indirective or too directive. Psychiatry has often caught the rebound from resentment because of a rather extreme indirect approach at times. However, Christian counselors have also been guilty at times of robbing the counselee of the benefit he could have gained in finding God's will for himself. Of course, there are many times to be directive. Discernment must be used to know which to use.

We believe the key here is *insight*. Once a counselee gains insight into the true nature of the problem, much of the problem may resolve.

Help the patient formulate a specific plan of action to deal with his problem. After one understands what a counselee's specific problems are, the next step is to help him formulate a plan of action. Although ventilating one's problems and expressing one's feelings of guilt and depression can be of much help, this alone is not enough. A specific plan of action is needed to deal with the problems and then, as problems are solved, feelings will change. Several counseling movements today (reality therapy, transactional analysis, and others) are stressing the importance of making specific plans and setting goals.

The Counseling Process

The counseling process could be understood as follows:

1. Let counselee *ventilate.* Listen to the counselee.

2. Help the counselee gain *insight.*

3. Work toward *emotional resolution* of the strong feelings emerging as the counselee deals with his insight into how the events and patterns of behavior have affected his life.

4. *Reprogram*—Help the counselee develop new, healthier "self-talk" and more productive patterns of behavior. Guide the patient toward opportunities to internalize a more balanced self-concept. Accountability and responsibility for one's choices play a key role here.

5. *Spiritual wholeness*—Assist the patient with scriptural insights, encouragement, and observations toward a deeper, more balanced, and healthier relationship with God.

This chapter has dealt in general with treating emotional problems. Previous chapters have dealt with recognizing spiritual, psychological, and physical problems. The following is an outline for ministers and Christian counselors of the counseling process for each of these three categories. One needs to remember that spiritual and psychological problems break down into four broad subdivisions, as in the following outline.

An Outline of the Treatment Measures for Spiritual, Psychological, and Physical Problems

I. Spiritual Problems (*see* 1 Thessalonians 5:14): Use one of five types of biblical counseling
   A. A need to know Christ (*see* Romans 1:16)
      1. During the course of counseling (after a relationship has been built), ask the counselee about his religious background.
      2. Share the Gospel.
      3. Write out verses on salvation (*see* Romans 3:23, 6:23; John 1:12).
      4. Keep it simple.
      5. Give counselee an opportunity to believe in Christ.

   B. A need to grow in Christ (*see* 1 Peter 2:2)
      1. Do a Bible study series with the counselee on discipleship. The Bible study should focus on the basics in the Christian life (God's Word, prayer, Christian fellowship, and witnessing). Help the counselee form a solid foundation in each of these areas and thus a balanced (healthy, mature) Christian life
      2. Have the counselee memorize three verses per week.
      3. Help the counselee figure out a specific plan for having a quiet time.
      4. Help the counselee become involved in a church. For further support, help the counselee become involved with a smaller group within the church (a minichurch).

   C. A need to deal with a specific sin (*see* 2 Thessalonians 3:5)
      1. Listen to the counselee and build a relationship.
      2. Confront the counselee about his sin
      3. Ask for a one-week commitment (until the next appointment) to avoid the sin.
      4. Give the counselee a short Bible study (approximately one page) on the problem area to do prior to the next

appointment. Make the focus of the Bible study on personal application.

5. Ask the counselee to memorize three verses per week that deal with the problem.

6. For support and strength to overcome the temptation, help the counselee to become involved with fellow Christians in a church, minichurch, or another Christian group.

7. Ask the counselee to have a quiet time daily.

D. Demonic influences (demon possession or demon oppression)

1. Share concepts in Ephesians 6.

2. Point out that Satan is aware of the particular temptations one is prone to and the weaknesses he has.

II. Psychological problems

A. Psychophysiologic problems (ulcer, colitis, high blood pressure, etc.)

1. Counsel with the counselee concerning the spiritual and psychological aspects of his problem.

2. Refer to the local medical doctor for treatment of the physical aspect of the problem.

3. If needed, work with another professional concerning the psychological aspect.

B. Personality trait or personality disorder

1. Discern the personality traits and vary your counseling approach accordingly. For example, do not approach an individual with hysterical traits the same as one with depression traits.

2. *Listen* with empathy as counselee tells of his presenting problem, past history, and feelings.

3. Explain to the counselee the strengths and potential weaknesses of his personality. Help him gain *insight*.

4. Help the counselee to formulate a specific *plan of action* to deal with his problem.

5. If needed, work with another professional who has training in psychology or psychiatry.

C. Depression, anxiety, and other major psychiatric disorders
    1. Discern the type of disorder and approach accordingly.
    2. *Listen* with empathy as counselee tells of his presenting problem, past history, and feelings.
    3. Explain to the counselee what he is doing and what is happening to him. Help him gain *insight*.
    4. Help the counselee formulate a specific *plan of action* to deal with his problem.
    5. If needed, work with another professional who has training in psychology or psychiatry. This may be needed when a threat of suicide or homicide exists. It will also be necessary when the counselor realizes the problem is beyond his ability to handle. If medication is needed, refer to a psychiatrist. If psychological tests are needed, refer to a psychologist. Of course, either can do therapy.

D. Psychosis (a loss of contact with reality)
    1. Work with another professional (local medical doctor, psychiatrist, or psychologist).
    2. Since the brain chemistry is usually altered in psychosis, medication is needed. Thus, the referral should be made to a psychiatrist.

III. Physical problems—Of course, physical problems will need to be referred to the local medical doctor or psychiatrist; but since spiritual and psychological factors may also be present, the counselor may wish to work with the doctor. The minister or layman should be especially alerted to the following physical problems that are often confused with psychological or spiritual problems.
    A. Hyperkinetic (hyperactive) child
    B. High or low blood-sugar levels
    C. Thyroid problems
    D. Organic brain syndrome of old age (senile dementia and Alzheimer's disease)
    E. Biochemical depression

The Decision-Making Process

A chapter on the principles of counseling and on treatment measures would not be complete without considering the decision-making process. Helping the counselee in the decision-making process is one of the key areas with which the counselor must deal. Individuals often ask how they can know if they are making the right decision. We believe the answer to this lies in examining three criteria. These are feelings, logic, and God's standard—the Bible. When we see individuals getting into trouble over faulty decisions, it is often because they are making their decisions according to feelings first, logic second, and God's Word last. Though feelings are the most unstable and the most unreliable of standards, many individuals run much of their lives on this basis. It is not uncommon to hear a husband or wife say that they are getting a divorce because they don't feel they love their mate anymore. When hearing this, one is reminded of the wise words of King Solomon when he stated that there was "a way that seemeth right unto a man but the end thereof are the way of death" (*see* Proverbs 14:12). Sadly, we have seen many individuals ruin their lives because they subjectively did what seemed in their feelings to be the thing to do.

More stable than feelings in making decisions is logic. This is simply considering the advantages and disadvantages of both sides of a decision and making the logical choice. Christians need to use this method more since many areas of decisions are not spoken of specifically in the Bible. We need to remember that God is the One who gives us our logic, and He wants us to use it. Of course, the danger with logic is that man is basically selfish, and without the guidance of the Holy Spirit, he will often choose a selfish course.

The best criterion for making decisions is God's Word. What is recorded in God's Word about a decision? Also related to God's Word is prayer, the conviction of the Holy Spirit, and advice from godly men.

10 Drugs Used in Psychiatry

Psychopharmacology in the Forefront

In the past, psychoanalysis has been the major thrust in psychiatry, but today psychopharmacology is coming to the forefront. Since many psychological problems have biological components and since the Lord usually works by natural means, I believe God is in agreement with the major asset that drugs have contributed to psychiatric therapy. An adequate knowledge of psychotherapeutic drugs can be of much practical importance to a Christian psychiatrist. In accordance with the upsurge of drug usage in psychiatry, the following discussion focuses on four problems often seen in psychiatry or general practice.

Schizophrenia

The term *schizophrenia* was made famous by Eugen Bleuler. In the early nineteen hundreds, he described the four A's that have come to be associated with schizophrenics. These are inappropriate affect, loose associations, ambivalence, and autistic thinking. He also, as other authors previously, had described the secondary symptoms such as hallucinations and delusions that may be present. We, too, have observed all these symptoms in patients and are convinced the condition termed *schizophre-*

nia exrsts largely as described m classical terms. For mstance, patients smile at circumstances that should have provoked a serious affect Patients ramble from one topic to another with no discernible connection The fear of patients responding to voices they heard incessantly has been observed. Arguments with individuals about their deeply ingrained delusions are futile These symptoms, consistent with a break with reality known as schizophrenia, are seen today as they were by Bleuler in the early nineteen hundreds

Bleuler made practical suggestions for the treatment of schizophrenia that are still applicable today.[1] However, today a group of drugs known as the major tranquilizers have revamped the therapy in schizophrenia. Chlorpromazine and reserpine were introduced as tranquilizers in 1954, and these drugs resulted in an upsurge of interest in psychopharmacology. On these or other major tranquilizers, most schizophrenics will improve. Of course, the amount of improvement varies with the individual. For instance, one lady was on the verge of a break with reality. She had not been sleeping, was having disturbing nightmares, and her speech indicated that distorted thinking was beginning. Because of major tranquilizers, this break was averted. Within a few weeks, she was sleeping well with no nightmares, and the disturbance in cognition had cleared.

The antipsychotic medications are called major tranquilizers or neuroleptics. Although their primary usage is for schizophrenia, other indications exist such as in paranoia, the manic phase of a manic-depressive illness, psychotic depressive disorder, and psychotic syndromes due to drug abuse such as cocaine or amphetamine intoxication. The most common side effects to the antipsychotic medications are extrapyramidal reactions and anticholinergic effects. Extrapyramidal reactions can include Parkinson-like symptoms, dystonias (muscle spasms and muscle contortions), and akathisia (a sense of restlessness or agitation in the muscles). The high-potency antipsychotic medications (e.g., Haldol, Prolixin, Stelazine) are more likely to produce extrapyramidal symptoms, whereas the lower-potency antipsychotic medications (e.g., Mellaril) have more anticholinergic effects (constipation, dry skin, dry mouth, blurred vision, and sometimes urinary retention). Severe anticholinergic symptoms can produce confusion and delirium. Tardive dyskinesia is a potential long-term hazardous side effect of antipsychotic medication that includes smacking of the lips, a chewing or rhythmic motion of the jaw, and a rolling or protruding in and out of the tongue. Sometimes there may be rhythmic twisting motions of the trunk or limbs as well. Although the disorder may onset after only a few months on the medications, it is much more commonly seen to occur after several years of use in generally high doses. Since it can be irreversible, the only generally accepted treatment for tardive dyskinesia is the cessation of antipsychotic medication when symptoms first occur.

Antipsychotic medications can cause other side effects such as increased sound sensitivity (chlorpromazine is sometimes a problem in this regard), jaundice, pigmentary retinopathy (a problem occasionally caused by thioridazine in doses over 800 milligrams per day), and periodically deposits of pigment in the skin or lens of the eye. Another potentially severe side effect to antipsychotic medications is neuroleptic malignant syndrome (NMS), which may develop with severe elevations in body temperatures, elevated pulse rate, and elevated muscle enzymes. A neuroleptic malignant syndrome does not appear to be directly related to a particular antipsychotic medication and may develop rapidly. It is a severe medical problem and needs to be aggressively treated by a qualified physician.

Unfortunately, all psychophrenic disorders and psychoses do not respond to the antipsychotic medications. In cases of treatment of refractory schizophrenia, a newer antipsychotic medication, clozapine, has been introduced and is showing some promising results. Clozapine (Clozaril, Sandoz) is intended for use only for patients who have failed to respond to at least two other less toxic therapies. Because of the risk of seizures and also agranulocytosis, close monitoring of the medication, along with regular white cell counts on a weekly basis, is necessary for its usage.

Depression

Because the rise in incidence of depression has been so rapid in America, the introduction of antidepressant medications in

1954 has proven to be of immeasurable value. Seventy percent of depressed patients are helped by antidepressant medications. We have personally seen patients respond with better moods, improved sleep, improved appetite, happier expressions, and an increased ability to concentrate, make decisions, and deal effectively with their problems. In clinical depression, there is often a biochemical defect. The exact mechanism of antidepressant medications is not fully understood, though there seems to be a significant effect on several areas of the brain, especially the limbic system, resulting in a down-regulation of post-synaptic beta receptors as the brain increases its supplies of serotonin and norepinephrine (serotonin and norepinephrine are key neurotransmitters in the brain that vitally affect the chemical balance of cognition and emotion). The proper use of antidepressant medications can be literally life-saving in individuals who are severely depressed. There is less and less confusion in the lay public about these medications, and thankfully there is much less stigma associated with the use of antidepressant medications than just one decade ago. These medications are not "chemical crutches," they are not addictive, they do not alter a person's identity, they do not diminish self-control, and they in no way encourage a person to avoid responsibility for his or her own decisions and actions. Surely no one would argue with giving a diabetic insulin. Then why should anyone argue with the utilization of a medication that causes the brain to be able to adjust itself back to the natural chemical balance with which it is designed to operate?

There are a variety of different antidepressant medications and various ways of classifying these. We propose four main classes of antidepressant medications: the first-generation (tricyclic) antidepressant medications, the second-generation (heterocyclic) antidepressant medications, the third-generation (bicyclic and unicyclic) antidepressants, and the MAO (monoamine oxidase) inhibitors. Imipramine was the first tricyclic antidepressant developed in the 1950s. Since then a variety of antidepressants have been implemented in this first-generation group of antidepressants, including amitriptyline (Elavil, Endep), nortriptyline (Pamelor, Aventyl), desipramine (Norpramine, Pertofrane), doxepin (Sinequan, Adapin), protriptyline (Vivactil), and trimipramine maleate (Surmontil). As far as it is understood at this point, these various antidepressants work similarly around the nervous system to correct the biochemical imbalance of depression. The choice of antidepressants is generally based on the particular profile of secondary side effects that may occur, such as blurred vision, orthostatic hypotension (dizziness), and weight gain.

The second-generation antidepressants include heterocyclic antidepressants, such as amoxapine (Asendin), maprotiline (Ludiomil), and trazodone (Desyrel). These antidepressant medications appear to work in generally the same fashion therapeutically as do the first-generation antidepressants. However, their side-effect profiles are somewhat different and, therefore, at times these medications may be particularly useful. The third-generation antidepressants such as the bicyclic compound fluoxetine (Prozac) and the unicyclic compound bupropion (Wellbutrin) are still newer antidepressants that have side-effect profiles that are by and large less problematic than either the first- or second-generation antidepressants. However, not any one patient responds equally well to all antidepressants and, therefore, the "fit" of an antidepressant medication to the individual patient can be somewhat difficult. Consequently, the professional attention of a psychiatric physician is frequently required.

The MAO inhibitors are also effective antidepressants. Medications such as phenelzine (Nardil) and tranylcypromine (Parnate) have been quite helpful in relieving depressions in patients who have simply not responded well to either the first-, second-, or third-generation antidepressant medications. Electroconvulsive therapy (ECT) can also be an effective treatment for severe depression and/or mania. This does require the application of electrical current to the patient's brain while the patient is under general anesthesia, and this treatment is generally recommended by psychiatrists only when the case is severe and treatment with appropriate medications is either impossible because of medical complications or has been given adequate trial and proved ineffective.

Concerning side effects, as mentioned above, the various antidepressants can cause anticholinergic drug symptoms, cardiac arrhythmias, and orthostatic hypotension, including jaundice, since the medications are generally metabolized in the liver. MAO inhibitors can cause a buildup of tyramine, which can cause a hypertensive crisis if excessive amounts of tyramine are ingested (such as in yeast, beans, beer, or cheeses).

The dosage of antidepressant medications is usually begun relatively low and then gradually built up, increasing the dose as tolerated about every third or fourth day. The antidepressant medications mentioned not only can be very effective for major depression but have also proven useful in many cases of panic attacks. Depressed patients receiving antidepressant medications may require from two to six weeks to show a full therapeutic response to the medication. Then, the medication is prescribed for generally six to eight months. At that point if clinical improvement is adequate, then a cautious tapering down of the medication can be prescribed under the monitoring of a physician. A majority of patients will be able to taper off the antidepressant without a relapse of the depression. More sophisticated laboratory monitoring methods have allowed the measuring of therapeutic blood levels of many of the antidepressants now, and this has proven helpful in assisting the physician in appropriately adjusting the dose of antidepressant medications.

Antianxiety

The group of medications commonly known to the public as "tranquilizers" are the antianxiety and sedative-hypnotics. They are also known as anxiolytics or minor tranquilizers. The first of these medications introduced in this country were the barbiturates, with other medications such as meprobamate (Equanil or Miltown) following. Librium and Valium are the two most widely known medications in the anxiolytic class. Their most effective role has been the short-term treatment of anxiety states and various psychological and physiological sequelae to anxiety Other medications used in the treatment of anxiety that fall into this class are clorazepate (Tranxene), lorazepam (Ativan), oxazepam (Serax), and alprazolam (Xanax) Antihistamine medications that have been shown to have some helpfulness in anxiety include hydroxyzine (Atarax and Vistaril).

Another new antianxiety medication, useful with some patients who have not responded to previous types of anxiolytic medications, is Buspirone (Buspar). This medication usually takes a bit longer for the antianxiety effects to be evident but is not thought to be habit forming. It cannot be used to treat withdrawal from the benzodiazepine family of antianxiety medications. One of the difficulties with the benzodiazepine antianxiety medicines is that they can be habit forming; and since they are anticonvulsant and sedative in nature, withdrawal from these medications can produce extreme agitation and seizures if done without medical supervision. The mode of action of the benzodiazepine medications is felt to be through enhancing activity of GABA receptors in the brain, the brain's own natural antianxiety regulating mechanism. In addition to this, the benzodiazepine alprazolam may have some effects on the noradrenergic system, causing some post-synaptic down-regulation of beta receptors and possibly increasing the activity of the N-protein (a protein that serves to help couple post-synaptic receptors to the intraneuronal energy system in the central nervous system of both).

Other medications used to down-regulate the noradrenergic system have included clonidine (Catapres) and propanolol (Inderal). These medications were generally developed for use in the cardiovascular system to regulate various cardiac and blood pressure conditions, but there has been usage of these medications in psychiatry in recent years for such problems as prevention of migraine headaches, panic disorder, reduction in neuroleptic-induced akathisia and the mitigation of withdrawal symptoms from opiates

Another category of sedative-hypnotic medications would be the medications used primarily as sleeping pills. There are several benzodiazepine medications that fall into this category, and these include primarily flurazepam (Dalmane), temazepam (Restoril), and triazolam (Halcion). These medications can be quite effective for the short-term relief of insomnia, but long-term use can produce physiological dependence on the medication, requiring a gradual and medically supervised withdrawal from the medication. Other medications used to assist with sleep have been the antihistamines diphenhydramine (Benadryl) and chlorhydrate (Noctec). Barbiturates and barbituratelike medications as well have been used for the short-term relief of insomnia, but these certainly must be monitored closely for the potential of abuse. These would include such medications as secobarbital (Seconal) and amobarbital (Tuinal), ethchlorvynol (Placidyl), and methyprylon (Noludar).

A medication that is not strictly a sedative, but certainly has been used in the treatment of alcoholism, is disulfiram (Antabuse), a drug that can be an effective assistant in the treatment of alcoholism. The patient taking disulfiram regularly will have an adverse reaction if alcohol is taken with the disulfiram. This is called the "alcohol-Antabuse" reaction and includes vomiting, sweating, blurred vision, rapid heart rate, rapid respiration, chest pain, and skin flushing. It is a very disconcerting reaction and can be dangerous if the reaction is severe, especially in patients with compromised physical health. Therefore, it is useful only in individuals who have a sincere desire to stop drinking and have an active involvement in an alcohol treatment recovery program.

Stimulants

The stimulant medications in psychiatry have largely included three medications: D-amphetamine (Dexedrine), methylphenidate (Ritalin), and magnesium pemoline (Cylert). These medications have been used by some physicians for suppression of appetite and by neurologists for the treatment of narcolepsy. In some cases, they may be effective as a short-term adjuvant in the treatment of depression

The most common use of the stimulant medications, especially Ritalin, has been for the treatment of attentional deficit disorder in children and adolescents. Children who are responding to the stimulant medication will rarely have any euphoria from the medication and in fact may be a bit sedated by the medication The positive effects that are hopefully achieved include improving the attention span, decreasing impulsivity and distractibility, and a more effective capacity to engage in organized behavior. The problems with stimulant medications can include addiction (such as addiction to D-amphetamine or methylphenidate) and the potential to induce psychotic reactions in some susceptible individuals. As mentioned, close and responsible medical management by a qualified professional for the use of these medications is indicated.

Medication Tables

Although the chart on the following page is quite technical, I believe it will prove of benefit to those in professional fields. It summarizes several authors' writings on drugs used in psychiatry.[2-8]

Drugs and Referrals

Because the field of psychopharmacology is very broad, the Christian counselor must not expect every physician to be closely acquainted with the effects and side effects of each and every drug available. Most physicians have an adequate knowledge of all the drugs. However, when a fine point of decision arises, he should trust the judgment of those psychiatrists who have specialized in the field.

Remember, the dosages and types of drugs mentioned in this chapter are not meant to be exact and are for academic use only. They are not intended to direct the use of any particular brand-named drug or treatment program. We would advise the patient seeking treatment to contact a qualified medical professional for individualized care.

Psychiatric Diagnosis: SCHIZOPHRENIA

Drugs	History of Drugs	*Approximate Dosages (in mg)/day			Side Effects
		Drug	Out-Patient Dosage	In-Patient Dosage	
Major Tranquilizers	1. Chlorpromazine and reserpine were introduced as tranquilizers in 1954.	1. Thorazine	30–400	400–1600	1. Drowsiness
1. Phenothiazines		2. Mellaril	50–400	75–800	2. Parkinson syndrome
a. Aliphatic		3. Stelazine	4– 10	6– 30	3. Allergic skin reactions
Thorazine		4. Prolixin	1– 3	2– 20	4. Hematologic disorders
b. Piperdine		5. Trilafon	8– 24	12– 65	5. Metabolic effects (as menstrual irregularities)
Mellaril		6. Navane	6– 15	10– 60	6. Restlessness
c. Piperizine		7. Haldol	2– 6	4– 15	7. Jaundice
Stelazine		8. Moban	20– 75	75–200	
Prolixin		9. Loxitane	20– 75	75–250	
Trilafon		10. Clozaril	(pending)		
2. Thioxanthene					
Navane					
3. Butyrophenone					
Haldol					
4. Molindone					
Moban					
5. Loxapine					
Loxitane					
6. Clozapine	Introduced February 1990				Clozapine must in addition be monitored closely for potential development of agranulocytosis and lowered seizure threshold
Clozaril					

*The dosages on this and following charts are not meant to be exact. Doctors needing details should refer to the *Physicians' Desk Reference*.

These charts are intended for academic use only. They are not intended to direct the use of any particular brand-named drug or treatment program.

183

Mode of Action of Major Tranquilizers

Phenothiazines are extremely active and have a wide range of biochemical reactions. Thus, it is difficult to know which reactions account for the desired effects. They affect parts of the brain as follows:

Cerebral cortex—not affected
Hypothalamus—inhibited
Reticular formation—inhibited
Limbic system—?
Thalamus—affects our neurotransmitters as dopamine
Neurotransmitter deposits—inhibited

Other Comments on Major Tranquilizers

1. These agents decrease anxiety.
2. They have antiemetic, antipruritic, and analgesic effects.
3. They do not produce tolerance.
4. They have beneficial effects on cognitive disturbances and perceptual changes that are characteristic of Schizophrenia.
5. When sedation is desired, Thorazine is an appropriate drug. When as little sedation as possible is desired, Stelazine is indicated.
6. In some conditions, one major tranquilizer may be recommended over others. If depression is also present in schizophrenia, some therapists use Mellaril. If agitation is prominent in schizophrenia, many therapists use Haldol. For obsessive-compulsive neurosis, some therapists try Haldol.
7. Phenothiazines may produce depression.
8. Phenothiazines are more effective than electric-shock therapy or psychotherapy in the treatment of schizophrenia.
9. Most patients improve. The amount of improvement varies.
10. The treatment of extrapyramidal side effects is with anticholinergics like Artane (2 mg 3x/day).
11. Mellaril may delay ejaculation.
12. Most phenothiazines can be given by mouth or intramuscularly.

Psychiatric Diagnosis: DEPRESSION—1. Sad facial expression, 2. Problem with sleep, 3. Decreased appetite, 4. Feelings of hopelessness and helplessness, 5. Feelings of guilt, 6. Anxiety.

Drugs	History of Drugs	*Approximate Dosage Range (mg/day)	Side Effects

I. First-generation antidepressants
  a. Imiprimine
    Tofranil,
    SK-Pramine
  b. Amitriptyline
    Elavil, Endep
  c. Doxepin
    Sinequan
  d. Nortriptyline
    Aventyl
  e. Desipramine
    Norpramine
  f. Trimipramine
    Surmontil
  g. Protriptyline
    Vivactil
	The prototype of the tricyclics was Tofranil. It was synthesized in 1954 and tested as a tranquilizer. It was accidentally found to have antidepressive activities.	Imipramine 150–300
		Amitriptyline 150–300
		Doxepin 150–300
		Nortriptyline 50–150
		Desipramine 150–300
		Trimipramine 150–300
		Protriptyline 15–60
			1. Tricyclics
			  a. Autonomic effects as dry mouth and difficulty in micturition
			  b. Cardiovascular effects as hypotension, tachycardia, and heart tracing changes
			  c. Endocrine effects as impotence, amenorrhea, decreased sex drive, and increased weight
			  d. Central nervous system effects as drowsiness, ataxia, and tremor
			  e. Hematologic disorders

Psychiatric Diagnosis: DEPRESSION (*cont.*)

Drugs	History of Drugs	*Approximate Dosage Range (mg/day)	Side Effects

II. Second-generation antidepressants
  a. Maprotiline
    Ludiomil
  b. Trazodone
    Desyrel
  c. Amoxapine
    Asendin
	These antidepressants have altered chemical structures of the core tricyclic structure.	Maprotiline 75–200
		Trazodone 150–600
		Amoxapine 150–400
			Generally these compounds have side effects similar to the first-generation compounds, but there are differences specific to various compounds.

III. Third-generation antidepressants
  a. Fluoxetine
    Prozac
  b. Bupropion
    Wellbutrin
	These antidepressants are unrelated to the first- and second-generation antidepressants chemically. Introduced in late 1980s.	Fluoxetine 20–60
		Bupropion 300–450
			These compounds are devoid of antihistamine and anticholinergic effects. They do not block alpha-1 receptors. Wellbutrin has certain use restrictions concerning seizure precautions.

IV. MAOI (monoamine oxidase inhibitors)
  a. Phenelzine
    Nardil
  b. Tranylcypromine
    Parnate
  c. Isocarboxazid
    Marplan
	The first MAOI, Iproniazid, was used in the treatment of tuberculosis and accidentally found to have antidepressant properties.	Phenelzine 45–90
		Tranylcypromine 30–50
		Isocarboxazid 30–50
			a. Similar to first-generation antidepressants
			b. Hypertensive crisis can be a complication.

186

Other Comments on Antidepressants

---

1. Approximately 70 percent of a depressed population are helped by antidepressants.
2. They do not produce tolerance. They are not addicting.
3. It takes one to two weeks for antidepressants to take effect.
4. Tricyclics are as effective if given in a single dose at bedtime.
5. Therapy should usually be given for six months.
6. Tofranil and Norpramin are probably used more than any other antidepressants.
7. If more sedation is desired to help a patient sleep better, Elavil is the drug of choice.
8. If the patient needs to be as alert as possible, Tofranil is the drug of choice.
9. Tofranil and Elavil are usually given by mouth but could be given intramuscularly.
10. Antidepressants should be used with caution in patients with increased intraocular pressure.
11. Tofranil will help in phobic reactions. MAOIs may help with panic disorder.
12. If a patient on MAOI should have a hypertensive crisis, he could be treated with Regitine (5 mg intravenously and repeated as needed).
13. Tofranil is the treatment of choice for bedwetting (enuresis).
14. Prozac has been effective with obsessive-compulsive symptoms associated with depression.

Psychiatric Diagnosis: ANXIETY

Drugs	History of Drugs	*Approximate Dosages (in mg)/day	Side Effects

Minor Tranquilizers
1. Benzodiazepines
  a. Chlordiazepoxide
    Librium
  b. Diazepam
    Valium
2. Propanediols—
  Meprobamate
  (Miltown)
  Hydroxyzine
3. (Vistaril)
	A large number of minor tranquilizers have been introduced in the last few decades.	1. Valium 5–60 mg/day
		2. Librium 15–100 mg/day
		3. Vistaril 25–200 mg/day
		4. Miltown 800–2400 mg/day
		5. Xanax 0.5–4 mg/day
		6. Ativan 1–4 mg/day
			Drowsiness
			Vertigo
			Increased appetite
			Headache
			Muscular weakness
			Impaired judgment
			Poor coordination
			Hypotension
			Bizarre behavior
			Menstrual irregularities

4. Buspirone (Buspar)		7. Buspar 10–30 mg/day	Buspar has a generally lower level of side effects, but the onset of action may be somewhat slower.

Mode of Action of Minor Tranquilizers

Their antianxiety effects are probably caused by their depressant influences on limbic structures; the benzodiazepines affect the GABA system.

They have a polysynaptic depressive effect that releases muscular spasms and thus muscular tension.

Other Comments on Minor Tranquilizers

1. They can produce tolerance.
2. They can be addicting.
3. They produce an immediate lift.
4. If minor tranquilizers are stopped abruptly, withdrawal symptoms may occur.
5. They should not be taken with alcohol.
6. Most minor tranquilizers can be given by mouth, intramuscularly, or intravenously.

Note: Several of the above comments are not expressly applicable to Buspar and Vistaril. (No medications should be taken with alcohol or drugs of abuse.)

Psychiatric Diagnosis: MANIC-DEPRESSIVE PSYCHOSIS

Drugs	History of Drugs	*Approximate Dosages (in mg)/day	Side Effects
Lithium Carbonate	Cade first reported beneficial effects in the manic phase of manic depressive psychosis in 1949.	Lithium can be started as low as 150 mg twice a day, but generally the daily dose must be increased to reach a therapeutic blood level of between 0.5 and 1.2 meq/liter.	"Drugged" feeling Fine tremor Drowsiness Muscular twitch Slurred speech Nausea, vomiting Diarrhea Central nervous system effects

Other Comments on Lithium

1. Initially, serum levels should be monitored daily. Later they can be monitored every one to three months.
2. Mania breaks usually in five to ten days on lithium.

3. Contraindications to lithium therapy are brain and renal damage. Caution should be used if the patient has heart damage
4. Lithium may cause diminished thyroid function over time.

Psychiatric Diagnosis: HYPERKINETIC CHILDREN
(Attentional Deficit Disorder)

Drugs	History of Drugs	*Approximate Dosages (in mg)/day	Side Effects
Ritalin Dexedrine Cylert	Amphetamines were developed in the late 1930s. All three of these drugs have shown to be more effective than placebo in the treatment of ADD (attentional deficit disorder).	Ritalin 5–60 mg/day Dexedrine 10–30 mg/day Cylert 37.5–75 mg/day	• Decreased appetite • Sedation in children (stimulation in adults) • Increased pulse rate is possible • Increased blood pressure is possible

Psychiatric Diagnosis: TRANSIENT INSOMNIA

Drugs	Approximate Dose at Bedtime	Side Effects
Dalmane	Dalmane 15–30 mg	• Sedation in A.M., "morning hangover"
Restoril Halcion Chloral hydrate	Restoril 15–30 mg Halcion 0.125–0.25 mg Chloral Hydrate 500 mg	• Slurred speech • Dizziness • Confusion (possibly paranoia, especially in the elderly) • Forgetfulness, usually associated with a sensation of being "overmedicated" • Dependence on the medication over time with rebound insomnia on withdrawal

More than that, I count all things to be loss in view of the surpassing value of knowing Christ Jesus my Lord.

PHILIPPIANS 3:8 NAS

I said, Days should speak, and multitude of years should teach wisdom. But there is a spirit in man: and the inspiration of the Almighty giveth them understanding. Great men are not always wise: neither do the aged understand judgment.

JOB 32:7–9

11 The Christian Counselor

A Letter From a Friend

Dr. Minirth relates a candid remembrance from his early days in medical training: "My first year of medical school had ended. Soon I would face the decision of whether or not to specialize in psychiatry. This was the setting when one morning I received a letter from a friend. The following is an excerpt from that letter.

Probably the most effective prayer you could pray at this time is that God would break our independency, pride, and selfishness (*see* 2 Corinthians 4:16–18). God grant (Leviticus 26:19) that we would as His children have a profound change in our personalities after this summer together with Him! I hear myself say, "I believe this, I believe that. . . ." I'm not too impressed with my beliefs if His words do not constitute my life and make a profound change in my relationship with my wife, children, other Christians, and people in general. Beloved God, give us the realization that we do not really have anything on this earth but Christ. The closest person to us is no longer ourselves but Jesus Christ who is our very life!

"I would later decide to go into psychiatry, and the principles laid down in that letter would further confirm in my mind the essential prerequisites for the character of a Christian counselor."

Five Key Characteristics

According to King Solomon, who penned Proverbs, Song of Solomon, and Ecclesiastes, a good counselor was a man who had wisdom and common sense. Solomon made reference to at least five characteristics that pertain to a wise man and, thus, certainly to one who hopes to help others find wisdom. These characteristics are: He is in pursuit of God (*see* Proverbs 9:10); he knows God's Word in a living way (*see* Proverbs 16:20, 22, 23); he knows the importance of prayer (*see* Proverbs 15:8); he values fellowship with godly people (*see* Proverbs 13:20); and he shares the Word of God (*see* Ecclesiastes 11:6).

In Pursuit of God

First, a wise man is one who hungers to know Christ more. Reflecting back on individuals we have known in the Christian life and through study in the Word of God, one theme resounds as the characteristic far above all others. That is the profound truth expressed by Apostle Paul when he wrote, "More than that, I count all things to be loss in view of the surpassing value of knowing Christ Jesus my Lord . . ." (Philippians 3:8 NAS). Paul was a man who utterly groaned to be more with Christ, to enjoy the sheer pleasure of His presence (*see* Philippians 1:21–24). Not only did Paul have this intense desire, but the same desire is found expressed over and over in the Old Testament, the New Testament, and by mighty men of God in more recent generations.

The Levites of the Old Testament days were priests chosen by the Lord for the specific purpose of ministering to Him. This reveals a very significant glimpse into the character of God and into what was in His heart—men who would be occupied much alone with Him. The New Testament continued with the same theme. It stated that we are priests chosen by God for the same purpose of showing His praise, thereby being impressed with Christ alone. There is no greater calling than to be occupied with Christ our Lord—not with what we are doing *for* Him, but *with* Him.

King David, probably one of the best known kings of all ages, is another example of an individual whose one desire in life was to know God intimately and behold His beauty (*see* Psalm 27:4). David said this was not one of many desires but his one desire. Thus, it is worth noting that the Lord said of David that he was a man after His heart. God used David to change the kingdom because of this trait and not because of David's abilities.

Apostle John recorded that God is actually seeking a particular type of man. The man God is seeking is the one who will be absorbed in really worshiping Him. Apostle John in John 4:23, 24 recorded that God seeks true worshipers who will worship Him in spirit and reality.

Edward M. Bounds, in his classic book *Power Through Prayer*, points out that the men who have accomplished the most for Christ were men who spent much time alone with Him. John Wesley spent two hours daily in prayer. Martin Luther spent at least two hours daily with the Lord. John Welch, a famous Scottish evangelist, spent eight hours a day with the Lord. In our lives we don't usually know a great many individuals whose greatest love and endeavor is to be intimately related to Jesus Christ. As counselors, such individuals tend to possess substantial wisdom and understanding. The lesson for us is perhaps best expressed by the modern-day author Aiden Tozer—Be in "pursuit of God."

The Bible is filled with the stories of such men. For example, Enoch was in pursuit of God. In Genesis 5:24 is recorded the following: "And Enoch walked with God: and he was not; for God took him." Also, Moses was in pursuit of God. In Exodus 33:11 is recorded that "And the Lord spake unto Moses face to face, as a man speaketh unto his friend." God looks for such men. In 2 Chronicles 16:9 is recorded, "For the eyes of the Lord run to and fro throughout the whole earth, to shew himself strong in the behalf of them whose heart is perfect toward him. . . ." The same is true today—*God is looking throughout the whole earth today for men in pursuit of Him.*

Growing Understanding of God's Word

A second characteristic of the man of wisdom is that he knows God's Word in a living way (*see* Proverbs 16:22, 23). This thought was expressed by Jeremiah when he stated, ". . . thy word was unto me the joy and rejoicing of mine heart . . ." (Jeremiah 15:16). Apostle Paul expressed the same ideal when he stated, "And now, brethren, I commend you to God, and to the word of His grace, which is able to build you up . . ." (Acts 20:32). The Lord Jesus Christ further expressed the importance of the thought when He stated, ". . . the words that I speak unto you, they are spirit, and they are life" (John 6:63). In recent times, God has used men such as Watchman Nee to express this concept that His Word is more than a documentary to be studied but is ". . . quick, and powerful, and sharper than any twoedged sword . . ." (Hebrews 4:12).

The Word of God not only instructs us, corrects us, and reproves us, but perhaps most of all, nourishes us. This is a concept that is often overlooked. Dr. Minirth relates the following personal example of this: "I never shall forget when I began to take the Scriptures as more than instructions and corrections but also nourishment and enjoyment. Through memorizing specific verses that met my needs, through praying God's Word back to Him, and through enjoying it with others, the Scriptures came alive to me."

God's words to us as recorded in the Bible by godly men not only provide us with spiritual nourishment but also protection in our age of spiritual and mental confusion. This age of confusion is one in which men base their eternal destinies on what others believe, while others believe many and varied things. What really matters is not what others believe, but what God's Word says! In the field of psychiatry there are many, many concepts. Some are simply not consistent with Scripture. Other concepts are helpful and do not disagree with Scripture. One of the best ways to evaluate concepts is by comparing them to the Word of God. Scripture memorization can be invaluable here. Not only has God's Word helped in evaluating concepts of mental health, but also the many and varied Christian views. A Christian without the Word of God memorized is open prey to the enemy and confusion of our day.

God's Word is not only helpful in evaluating others, but it has been an equally valuable source to evaluate whether thoughts and conflicts within our lives have been merely of ourselves or of God. In Hebrews 4:12 Apostle Paul recorded, "For the word of God is quick, and powerful, and sharper than any twoedged sword, piercing even to the dividing asunder of soul and spirit, and of the joints and marrow, and is a discerner of the thoughts and intents of the heart." Thus, the Word of God helps us distinguish between "soulish" issues (those coming merely from ourselves) and spiritual issues.

In conclusion, since there are so many books on counseling and psychology to which we may turn for help, we might do well to remind ourselves as did King Solomon when he stated, "The words of the wise are as goads, and as nails fastened by the masters of assemblies, which are given from one shepherd. And further, by these, my son, be admonished: of making many books there is no end; and much study is a weariness of the flesh" (Ecclesiastes 12:11, 12). By analogy, we will do well to remind ourselves of the importance of God's Word over even many books of psychiatry and psychology, though these can be helpful.

When considering the effect of God's Word upon our lives, it is important to note that anything so deeply held as one's faith and one's confidence in the Scriptures can affect the unconscious mind. Scientific data have shown the importance of the unconscious mind. A neurosurgeon named Wilder Graves Penfield found out that by touching electrodes to different areas of the brain, individuals were able to remember specific past events and the feeling that went along with the event.[1] It was found that current-day events often trigger feelings of the past without the event itself being recalled. Thus, an individual may hear a song and feel sad but not know why he feels sad until later, when he remembers how the song related to a past event.

Feelings of rejection often relate more to past events than to the current-day situation. For example, a man feared being rejected by others, although few current-day events could explain those feelings. In therapy, it was discovered he feared rejection by others when he was young. Now, the least event could trigger these feelings. It was as though a tape of these feelings of the past were being replayed. Of course, not only may the feelings of the past be replayed, but the actual event may be remembered also. Also, the old event may be recalled without a clear-cut current triggering event.

In any event, all of this simply says that the unconscious mind is an important factor in conscious behavior, and significant events that have been recorded by the brain do affect present behavior. This speaks to the tremendous importance of saturating our minds with the knowledge of the Word of God. As the Word of God is enjoyed and memorized, it sinks into the subconscious and is there for years to come. It can be a significant determinant of behavior. David expressed it this way:

> Wherewithal shall a young man cleanse his way? by taking heed thereto according to thy word.

> Thy word have I hid in mine heart, that I might not sin against thee.

> PSALM 119:9, 11

All of the above points to the fact that the Word of God can be of immeasurable power in our lives. Dr. Minirth puts some perspective on this with the following anecdote from the early days of the clinic. "Recently I was meditating on Hebrews 11:3, 'Through faith we understand that the worlds were framed by the word of God, so that things which are seen were not made of things which do appear.' The words contained in that verse encouraged me to do research on the power of God's Word. I found that if one traveled at the speed of light (186,000 miles per second), he would be 100,000 years old if he traveled across the diameter of the Milky Way.[2] Furthermore, there are several hundred billion galaxies like the Milky Way. My mind could hardly comprehend the size of the universe. And then I thought, *If God created the universe by His Word, then what could His Word do in my life?*"

Understands the Power of Prayer

Prayer makes the realities of God's Word personal. It can give us insight into how to share insights and applications with our counselees. A third characteristic of a godly counselor is, therefore, that he knows the importance of prayer. A danger in Christian counseling is a total reliance upon methods rather than God's power made possible through prayer. God uses methods, and much can be learned didactically that aids in counseling. However, our methods are always secondary in importance to God's healing power. Accordingly, James recorded that Elias was a godly man but was ". . . subject to like passions as we are, and he prayed earnestly . . ." (James 5:17). To be sure, more can be accomplished by prayer than we ever dream possible.

Prayer is communion with God. This communion is possible because of Christ's death for us and because of His indwelling Holy Spirit. Effective prayer is only possible through a relationship with God through Christ. Once that relationship has been established by placing faith in Christ, God longs for us to talk with Him. In Proverbs, Solomon recorded that God delights in our prayers (*see* Proverbs 15:8).

Prayer may consist of praise (*see* Psalm 9:11), confession (*see* 1 John 1:9), or thanksgiving and supplication (*see* Philippians 4:6).[3] Confession relieves us of our sense of guilt. Being thankful is an encouragement to both us and our gracious Father. Supplication can accomplish unlimited means as it gives God the opportunity to either answer our primary request or the desire in the request. But the prayer that we have found the most helpful of those above is praise. In praise we become absorbed in someone other than ourselves. Many problems can be the result of self-involvement. Praise can remedy this. Moses became so discouraged when he was self-involved with his eyes on self rather than God that he wanted to die. His prayers indicated self-concern more than God-concern. Christ also pointed to priority when He stated, "But seek ye first the Kingdom of God" (*see* Matthew 6:33). This applies to our prayers as well, lest our very prayers become self-centered. Singing songs to the Lord or praying His words of praise back to Him can be of utmost *practical* importance for mental as well as spiritual health.

We have found several helpful "how to's" concerning prayer. Practicing prayer is the most important of all. We must "exercise" our spirits to do it. Then God will gradually teach us important applications and wonders of prayer. It is recorded in the Bible that Moses talked with God as a friend to a friend. This kind of deep prayer relationship developed primarily because Moses simply talked much with God. To be sure, Moses initially could not know all of the various aspects of prayer, but he knew God as his friend as well as his God and felt free to talk with Him. God longs for us to consider Him a friend and to talk with Him and call upon Him during moments throughout the day. I believe this is the most important "how to."

Fellowship with Godly Men and Women

A fourth characteristic of wise counselors is that they know the importance of fellowship with godly men and women. In Proverbs 13:20 Solomon recorded, "He that walketh with wise men shall be wise. . . ." Further, in Proverbs 27:17 Solomon recorded, "Iron sharpeneth iron; so a man sharpeneth the countenance of his friend." The wise King Solomon continued with the same theme in Ecclesiastes when he wrote, "Two are better than one; because they have a good reward for their labour. For if they fall, the one will lift up his fellow; but woe to him that is alone when he falleth; for he hath not another to help him up" (Ecclesiastes 4:9, 10). It is interesting to note that together the condition of falling is only a *possibility* but alone it is almost a *certainty*.

Fellowship with godly individuals has taught both of us much about counseling both from a didactic view as well as practical experience. From others, we have learned techniques: We have learned to listen; we have learned the importance of keeping confident what others relate; but most of all, we have gained by being exposed to the measure of the grace of Christ in their lives.

A Witness for Christ

Finally, the wise counselor is one who sows the Word of God. He is one who testifies of Christ to others both by his actions and his words. God promises to bless His Words (*see* Isaiah 55:11) and not our words. Whether an individual allows this Word to prosper for him is his responsibility, but our job is to share it in an appropriate manner. By analogy, if not by direct implication, we can learn a lesson from King Solomon who wrote, "In the morning sow thy seed, and in the evening withhold not thine hand; for thou knowest not whether shall prosper, either this or that, or whether they both shall be alike good" (Ecclesiastes 11:6). A counselor is responsible to share God's Word and His guidance.

Qualities of a Christian Counselor

In addition to the basic characteristics reflective of the character and life-style of a Christian counselor, there are also certain overall qualities that are vital for him or her to acquire. To a degree, these qualities can be learned, but we believe that crucial to their expression is the work of the Holy Spirit flowing through the Christian counselor. The following are a sampling of ten such qualities that we believe are significant.

1. Have an Accepting Attitude

One quality that a counselee needs in a counselor is an attitude of acceptance. Problems are normal, and no one is above them. We have heard others imply that their fellow Christians should not have problems, but little do they realize that this is one of the major means God uses to conform us to His image. Ministers and deacons have problems just as everyone else, but they may feel ashamed to share their problems or may feel that no one would accept that they, too, need understanding and counsel. We all have problems, and God desires that we accept and counsel one another. It is often the case that we really begin to grow rapidly spiritually when we find a couple of other brothers or sisters in Christ who accept us with no conditions.

2. Be a Good Listener

A second quality of a godly counselor is that he is a good listener. He listens with interest and without fidgeting or hurrying. He listens without interruptions and shows warmth through the expression of his eyes. Further, a good listener allows the person to finish sharing what he perceives his problem to be before helping him gain insight. He uses properly inserted questions that initially are used to obtain information and clarify issues but can later be used to provoke thinking and help the counselee reach his own conclusions. Elihu, a counselor in Old Testament times, knew the importance of listening when he stated, "Behold, I waited for your words, I listened to your reasonings, While you pondered what to say. I even paid close attention to you . . ." (*see* Job 32:11, 12 NAS). Many are willing to speak, but few are willing to listen.

3. Be Suggestive and Confronting When Appropriate

A third quality of a godly counselor is that he knows how to give suggestions. There is a time for suggestive statements, and often these will be received when a statement would be rejected. We have found suggestive phrases helpful at the opportune time, whereas a good counselor also knows when to be direct and confronting. In Proverbs 27:6 is recorded the following, "Faithful are the wounds of a friend. . . ."

In summary, there are times to be suggestive, and times to be confronting. The good counselor can discern which to use.

4. Interject Scripture

A fourth quality of the godly counselor is that he knows how and when to interject Scripture. Proper timing and readiness are important. Once the counselee knows the counselor really cares, Scripture can usually be shared without any offense. The Scripture must meet the specific need of the individual, and a few verses are preferable to many. Likewise, we have found it helpful to copy the verses down for the counselee. At the appropriate time, prayer with a counselee is also of great benefit.

5. Use Proper Attitude

A fifth quality that is helpful is discerning the right attitude to employ to help various personalities. Various attitudes are:

matter-of-factness, firm kindness, active friendliness, and passive friendliness. Christ was often matter-of-fact, and yet He knew when to use firm kindness or another attitude. A counselor might use a matter-of-fact attitude with a brother living in sin, firm kindness with a depressed brother, active friendliness with those who really want and need encouragement, and passive friendliness with those who have paranoid trends. Each person is different, and by being sensitive to his spirit, the counselor can employ an attitude to which the counselee can best respond.

6. Have an Unwavering Purpose for Christ

A sixth quality of a Christian counselor is an unwavering purpose for Christ. There are thousands of individuals today who are looking for someone with a purpose for living—someone who knows where he is heading—someone who is living for Christ.

7. Be Personal

Counselees need counselors who are warm, open, honest, genuine, and very personal. To be open and honest themselves, they must sense the same from the counselor. They want to sense that the counselor is personally interested in them and their problems. As has been pointed out by William Glasser, most who need psychiatric help have not been able to fulfill two basic needs in life—love and self-worth.[4] A warm, personal counselor can be one person who can give them love and self-worth. The Scriptures repeatedly point to the need to be personal (*see* Galatians 4:19; Proverbs 12:25; Philippians 1:3–8).

8. Be Unshockable

A young man recently commented, "I could never have shared these things with Reverend Q." He went on to indicate how shocked his minister would have been. A good counselor does not act shocked upon hearing a counselee's story. This only frightens the counselee, prevents him from sharing the guilt he may so need to share, and prevents him from learning how to deal with it effectively. Christ was not shocked with the problems of men for ". . . he knew what was in man" (John 2:25). When Christ was helping the woman of Sychar (*see* John 4), he did not seem shocked at her past. He dealt with it straightforwardly and effectively.

9. Be Confident

A good counselor offers the counselee realistic hope. He is confident in Christ, in his ability as a counselor through Christ, and in what Christ can accomplish in the counselee. If we think we can help a person, we let him know it. If we think a depressed person will start feeling better, we tell him so. We try to offer what we consider to be realistic hope. We do try to be realistic. For example, we would not tell a person with an I.Q. of 80 that we felt he could go to college. Rather, we would help him make realistic plans. In Hebrews 10:35, 36 is recorded, "Cast not away therefore your confidence, which hath great recompense of reward. For ye have need of patience, that, after ye have done the will of God, ye might receive the promise."

10. Have a Sense of Humor

A counselor needs a sense of humor. He deals with many serious problems daily; and without a sense of humor, the load can be too much. He needs at times to be able to help his counselee have this same sense of humor. For example, we have found that obsessive-compulsive people often begin to improve when they can start to laugh at their perfectionism.

Seven Therapeutic Steps in Christian Counseling

At the Minirth-Meier Clinic, we believe that seven steps are important to the counselor in providing therapy to the client. They are as follows:

1. Be kind

Proverbs 19:22 states that what is desirable in a man is kindness. The Apostle Paul in 1 Thessalonians 2:7 tells us that we should be "gentle." Furthermore, scientific research in evaluating different psychotherapeutic approaches found that it is not so much the specific approach used in therapy, as the specific therapist. Therapists who exude warmth and genuineness and who are empathetic are the ones who get good results. Also, consider how warm the Apostle Paul was toward those he was helping (Galatians 4:19; Philippians 1:7). Showing kindness is one of the most important principles of all. A person cannot hear you if he or she does not sense that you care for them.

2. Start with behavior

Often, an important starting point in therapy is a focus on behavior. While therapy certainly involves much more, this is nonetheless an important step. When Solomon, the wisest man who ever lived (other than Christ), was giving the essence of the responsibility of man, one of his two areas of recommendation had to do with behavior (Ecclesiastes 12:13). The Scriptures are replete with emphases on behavior, from Genesis 4:6, 7 throughout the rest of the Bible. The importance is magnified in verses such as Philippians 2:13, "For it is God which worketh in you both to will and to do of his good pleasure" and in Philippians 4:13, "I can do all things through Christ which strengtheneth me," as well as through the entire Book of James.

Also, it is important to realize that although feelings are extremely important and should be listened to, most individuals have very little direct control over changing their feelings. In my years of practice, I have rarely seen a depressed individual feel sad and choose immediately to feel happy. What we do have control over, however, is behavior. We choose what time we get up, whom we talk with during the day, whether or not we exercise, whether or not we read and study the Scriptures, and so on. We have maximum control over what we do. We each tend to follow a cycle where feelings follow behavior and behavior follows feelings. Let's interrupt where we have control—in the area of behavior. We often start by having patients make a specific behavioral plan involving daily quiet time, weekly exercise programs, daily social contact, and avoiding specific sinful behaviors (Proverbs 4:12). Helping to redirect behavior also gives the new client a feeling of direction and control. To just be listened to and then left to oneself without clear guidelines is often very disturbing for the client.

3. Help the client gain insight

King David stated this principle very clearly in Psalm 139:23, 24: "Search me, O God, and know my heart: try me, and know my thoughts: And see if *there be any* wicked way in me, and lead me in the way everlasting." The Apostle Paul wrote the epistles to educate the churches and to help them gain insight into their behavior. If you evaluate it from a scientific standpoint, then you would come to this conclusion: One cannot change if one does not know the problem. If a religious leader thinks his demanding perfectionism or his unwarranted suspicions and paranoia come from godliness, how can he change? If a husband thinks his use of Ephesians 5:22 to make his wife more submissive is based on godliness, when he in reality may be very selfish, how can he change? If a Christian leader's relentless drive comes from past issues, and he is really addicted to an excessive work schedule in the cloak of having a successful ministry for Christ, how can he change? Indeed, knowing how the past affects the present and creates sinful defense mechanisms, which turn into ungodly transference issues and then into inappropriate injunctions, is an invaluable tool.

How can a person change, if he does not know what the problem is?

4. Help with the resolution of feelings

Dr. Paul Meier, our friend and business partner for many years, has made the comment that hurt feelings and bitterness not dealt with become like a festering sore. When lancing the sore, pain is elicited, but if the sore is not lanced, disease results. Clients do need to be honest about their feelings. To deny feelings does not make them go away. God knows everything; He knows how we feel. Years of repressing the feelings resulting from a history of abuse in early life does not make them go away. Feelings are recorded in biochemical pathways of the brain, and they cannot be simply erased. They have to be resolved by using kindness and by reprogramming them through the use of Scripture (Psalm 119:9–11) and through being around others in the body of Christ. To tell a Christian he shouldn't have certain feelings when they do exist is not being honest. Better to say, "I understand how you feel. Let's see what would be a godly approach to dealing with that feeling; and by all means let's be honest about it." It has been said that to be listened to is one of the most moving experiences in life. Also, we can remind ourselves of the saying that a burden shared is only half a burden. To allow a person to share true feelings is only common sense, and to understand is only kind.

5. Help them to reprogram their thinking

We do not believe, as many behavioral therapists do, in the simple theory that a stimulus produces response. We believe that between the stimulus and response lies the individual's belief system. The importance lies not just in what happens to us in life, it is what we believe about what happens to us—our belief system. For example, the Christian should not view death as a non-Christian would.

Life is tough at times, but the Christian's whole belief system can alter how he views life and can program his feelings and his physiological and behavioral response (2 Corinthians 4:16–18). Romans 12:2 encourages us to be transformed by the renewing of our minds. Philippians 4:8 alerts us to being aware of our way of thinking. It is also easy for the Christian to personalize, magnify, and overgeneralize issues to focus on some minute detail without seeing the big picture. It is easy for us to make ourselves miserable wanting everyone's love and approval, when God's love should be our satisfaction. It is easy for the Christian to feel that his unhappiness is externally caused and not to remind himself that Christ can make a huge difference. It is easy for the Christian to have beliefs that simply are not true (e.g., "God won't forgive me!" "God could never use me; I'm too weak!").

In some respects, the mind could be compared to a huge computer, perhaps about the size of the Pentagon, with miles and miles of tapes. When new data are being evaluated, the mind scans through this vast library of tapes in search of knowing what kind of behavior, feeling, and physiological response to give. Our therapists claim the theory that the Christian can reprogram these tapes through the Word of God and through input by other Christians. Utilizing these tools can make a world of difference in the person's outlook on life. Consider the impact that the following verses could have on this concept: Deuteronomy 32:46,47; Joshua 1:8; Psalm 1:2,3; Jeremiah 5:14; Isaiah 40:8; Matthew 24:35; John 15:7; Luke 24:32; John 6:63; 2 Timothy 3:16,17; 1 Thessalonians 2:13; Hebrews 11:3; and 1 John 2:14.

6. Use a comprehensive and balanced approach along with good common sense

The approach should be comprehensive. What a sin to do therapy with someone for three years and then to realize you have been counseling a brain tumor. Medical disease should always be ruled out first. How one feels is extensively dependent on one's medical condition. Man is one being—spirit, soul, and body. When we affect one part, we invariably affect the other two. The medical, psychological, and spiritual should all be considered. Indeed, the approach should be comprehensive.

Second, the approach should be balanced. For example, to ignore the spiritual aspect is to forget what really counts in life—that is, where one spends eternity. It is to forget that the secular schools have no standard of authority, such as the Bible. It is to forget that willpower can be ineffective (Romans 7:18). It is to forget that man is basically selfish (Jeremiah 17:9). It is to forget that the Scriptures are not locked into any one specific approach—behavioral, cognitive, or insight oriented. The Scriptures are broad, and they are balanced.

To overemphasize the psychological is to forget that the non-Christian cannot understand the spiritual (1 Corinthians 2:14). The other extreme is ignoring the psychological altogether and doom some to a life of psychosis and others to death. It is to ignore scientific knowledge in one field of medicine (psychiatry), while accepting it in other areas, such as internal medicine. It is to realize that many psychological problems have a medical aspect and to come across to a watching secular world as being ignorant and extreme.

To ignore the psychiatric problems is to not realize that a significant part of psychiatry is medical. I recall one missionary sent to us because she was "lazy." In reality, she had a brain tumor. I also recall a seminary student who came to us with psychosis. His church pulled him out of treatment because they thought it was a spiritual problem. Of course, his behavior had spiritual and psychological dimensions; but there was also a base problem with the neurotransmitters within his brain. To ignore psychiatry altogether is not using common sense.

Third, a therapeutic approach should involve good common sense. I define this as knowing how to apply wisdom in day-to-day living. I recall one Christian counselor who became enthralled with one specific approach. He lost common sense when it came to helping people deal with feelings and became emotionally and physically involved with his clients, rationalizing in his mind that he was helping them. This is a traumatic example of the loss of common sense, but there are many more subtle areas to which we could refer. We need to strive in Christian counseling to avoid extremes and use common sense in all areas.

7. Remember the importance of the spiritual

Although man is comprehensive, indeed, the spiritual is the most important aspect of all. Eternity is forever. How could anyone overemphasize how important it is to know Christ and to spend eternity with Him? To help someone solve their earthly problems and then ignore where he would spend eternity is useless. Furthermore, although individuals can be helped without knowing Christ, He is an unbelievable power source in overcoming any spiritual or psychological problem. Although we do not understand it, we believe that Jesus Christ deeply enjoys spending time with us. To know Him, enjoy Him, to have a best friend in Him is the most powerful resource on earth. Enoch must have felt some of this in Genesis 5:24, where we read that "Enoch walked with God. . . . " Also, Moses must have felt some of this in Exodus 33:11, where it says, "And the Lord spake unto Moses face to face, as a man speaketh unto his friend. . . ."

It is our prayer as Christian counselors that we may know Christ, walk with Him, let Him fill our inner being; and, indeed, we will be able to help others because He is living in us.

Much can be learned from godly
counselors of the past. Although not
applying directly to Christian counselors, Paul said, ". . . join in following my example.   . ."
PHILIPPIANS 3:17 NAS

12   Four Biblical Counselors

One of the best methods of learning how to counsel effectively is
to study men of the past who were skilled in this field. Two
counselors from Old Testament days and two from New Testament days offer significant guidance in the field of counseling.
Solomon and Elihu come to us from the Old Testament; Christ
and the Apostle Paul are examples from the New Testament.

Elihu

The record of Elihu's counseling occupies six chapters in the
Book of Job, thus Elihu is one of the earliest godly counselors
recorded by God. Although Elihu is not well known, he demonstrated much in the way of wise counsel, and little in the way
of poor counsel. Thanks to Elihu, we can learn much from his
mistakes.

Job was a friend of Elihu's. Job was a godly man, but Satan
argued that Job was godly because of the benefits he had received. Satan was granted permission from God to try Job with
suffering. Job began to suffer much physically and mentally. He
lost his health, his wealth, and his family. Four friends of Job's
came to counsel with him concerning his condition. Initially all
four did well. They just listened, and Job must have greatly

benefited from their company. Then the first three counselors made their mistakes.

The first three counselors were Eliphaz, Bildad, and Zophar. These counselors made four significant errors. First, they proved to be talkers, and not listeners. They had some true and eloquent advice, but the advice was not practical. They were too directive, too fast. They were legalistic and dogmatic. Second, they failed to convey an attitude of paramount importance. They were not understanding but, rather, harsh and cruel. They were accusers, not counselors. Third, their discourses are filled with evidences of pride, and pride is downfall to any counselor. Finally, they had an inadequate concept of God. They saw God as being petty in His relations with man and failed to see the glory, grace, and mercy of God. These four errors accounted for their failure as counselors and will account for failure among counselors today.

Elihu was different from the other counselors. He was much younger. He was a better listener. He was polite, sincere, and honest. He indicated depth in his thinking. He had a higher concept of God. He knew the importance of expressing himself, but at the appropriate time. Some quotes from and about Elihu are:

Now Elihu had waited to speak to Job because they were years older than he.

JOB 32:4 NAS

I said, Days should speak, and multitude of years should teach wisdom. But there is a spirit in man: and the inspiration of the Almighty giveth them understanding. Great men are not always wise: neither do the aged understand judgment.

JOB 32:7–9

Lo, all these things worketh God oftentimes with man, To bring back his soul from the pit, to be enlightened with the light of the living.

JOB 33:29, 30

I will fetch my knowledge from afar, and will ascribe righteousness to my Maker.

JOB 36:3

Although Elihu also committed errors, God did not rebuke him
as He did the other three counselors when He stated, ". . . My
wrath is kindled against thee, and against thy two friends: for ye
have not spoken of me the thing that is right . . ." (Job 42:7). In-
cidentally, God was merciful to the three counselors even though
they were wrong, and He accepted Job's prayer in their behalf.

Additional comments on the counseling of Elihu have been
made by Scofield.[1]

Solomon

Of all the men mentioned in the Bible with the exception of
Christ, Solomon outranks them all as a counselor. Solomon is a
counselor's counselor. His therapeutic approach is directive. His
counseling approach could be very directive because his counsel
agreed with the counsel of God. In fact, God gave Solomon's
writings on counseling more merit than any other. Nowhere else
in the Bible is such length and detail on counseling written as in
Proverbs. The Book of Proverbs contains the secrets to a wealth
of wisdom. In this book, Solomon covered such topics as rules
for mental health, descriptions of sociopaths, descriptions of the
hysterical woman, the road to wisdom, characteristics of the
wise, and rules for raising children. Solomon dealt very specifically with these and other issues, and we have been impressed
with the similarity between his descriptions of certain conditions
and that described in psychiatric texts.

The Book of Proverbs may be compared with two other books
also written by Solomon—Song of Solomon and Ecclesiastes. In
Ecclesiastes, Solomon described his search for meaning in life.
He tried wealth, sex, humanitarian efforts, and intellectual pursuit. His conclusion was "Vanity of vanities . . ." (Ecclesiastes
1:2). In Song of Solomon, Solomon wrote a love story. If one
abstracts somewhat, he may consider this an analogy of the love
Christ has for each one of His children and the resulting fulfillment that one finds in Christ alone. Watchman Nee in his book
Song of Songs has so aptly contrasted the "vanity of vanities"
conclusion in Ecclesiastes with the "song of songs" conclusion in
the Song of Solomon (*see* Song of Solomon 1:1). Thus, in Song of

Solomon, God has revealed the beginning of wisdom. The beginning of wisdom is to be in pursuit of a deep relationship with Jesus Christ. In Proverbs the expanse of that wisdom is broadened into abundant practical advice.

Jesus Christ

Although Solomon was the wisest man who ever lived, he was not the wisest counselor. That distinction belongs to One who was not only man but also God—Jesus Christ. Jesus Christ was the Counselor of counselors. There are six areas in which He excelled in counseling.

The Lord Jesus Christ had perfect insight into a man's problem. Insight is of paramount importance in helping others in counseling. The therapist must have insight into what the real problems are, and he must be able to help the patient gain this insight. Christ could do both of these.

As stated previously, Christ was an expert at asking questions. He used questions to teach, to help others gain insight, and to rebuke irresponsible behavior. The ability to use questions in a counseling situation is an act of invaluable measure.

Third, Christ really cared for those He counseled. This is something people can sense. It is something innate that we can usually read in others. Really caring for a person accounts for much of his improvement. Most people with emotional problems have had difficulty finding others they can relate to and who give them a feeling of self-worth. Christ knew how to be matter-of-fact, rebuking, or friendly; and yet, He could relate that He really cared.

Fourth, Christ could counsel others because of His close relationship with God the Father. This is a prerequisite to doing Christian counseling. Someone who walks and talks with God knows himself, his weaknesses, and his strengths through God. He understands man and has insight into problems. He has available to him the wisdom of God. How can one help others learn to live if he does not know himself? Christ knew the Word of God. In fact, He *was* the Word of God. The Word of God and the relationship with God developed through the Word, and prayer forms the foundation of Christian counseling.

Christ understood a man's problems. He knew what the man needed to do to change and deal with his problems. And, finally, He knew how to motivate the man to change. Christ could help an individual formulate a plan of action to deal with his problems.

The sixth reason Christ excelled in counseling was His balance. He knew when to be overtly directive and when to ask questions to help the person gain insight. He knew when something that happened to an individual in the past needed to be dealt with and when to deal with the here and now. Christ knew the importance of feelings and how to focus on needed behavioral changes. In both Christianity and psychiatry, there is often a trend toward extremes; Christ had perfect balance.

Apostle Paul

There is one individual who should be mentioned as an example of Christian counselors because it was he and not Sigmund Freud who first wrote concerning the psychic forces that play on the mind of man. Apostle Paul, writing to early Christians, explained that their minds would be drawn between an old nature and a new nature and that they could choose what to do in each case. The analogies are not exact, but similar. The *id* would correspond to the old nature. The *superego* would correspond to the new nature (indwelling Christ), or the conscience of a non-Christian. The *ego* would correspond to the will. However, Paul goes even deeper into the makeup of man and talks about a body, a soul (consisting of a mind, emotion, and will), a spirit, the flesh, a good but weak law of the mind, an evil law of the members, a supreme law of the Spirit, an external deadening law, and how all of these parts interrelate (*see* Romans 6, 7, and 8; Hebrews 4:12; 1 Thessalonians 5:23; and 1 Corinthians 4:16). There are indeed some similarities between the writings of Sigmund Freud and the teachings of the Apostle Paul, but there is no doubt that Paul has the scriptural answers.

Ministers face a difficult problem in deciding if, when, and how to refer to a professional.

THE AUTHORS

13 Professional Help—When and How to Refer

Is this a spiritual problem or a mental problem? Should I refer this counselee to a psychiatrist? Will the psychiatrist take away the client's faith in God?

The above are typical questions that ministers ask. They are valid questions. Below are given some guidelines on when to refer to another professional.

If the client is suicidal or homicidal, then the minister should refer. The counselee may need immediate hospitalization to prevent him from harming himself or others. Such statements as "Life doesn't seem worth living"; "I wish I were dead"; and "Everything seems hopeless" indicate suicidal thoughts and plans. The counselee should be asked if he has had suicidal thoughts, plans, or attempts. If he has, he should be referred. Likewise, the counselee should be asked about any desires to harm others. If he has any, then, again, he should be referred.

If a person has lost contact with reality, then he should be referred. He may have delusions (as a fear that the Mafia is after him), or he may be having hallucinations (seeing or hearing things not present). These individuals often misinterpret whatever is said to them, and counseling alone is usually not effective. With medication, plus counseling, a chronic mental case may be prevented, and the counselee can be restored to reality.

If a counselee is extremely euphoric, has pressure of speech, and is extremely hyperactive, he may be manic. There seems to be a genetic and chemical abnormality here, and dramatic results can be obtained with a drug known as lithium. With the drug, most counselees return to normal. Without the drug, the counselee is dangerous to himself, makes extremely poor judgments that can result in financial failure, and is impossible to counsel. Such a patient needs referral to a professional.

Another problem with an organic base that needs referral is the hyperkinetic reaction (attention deficit disorder) of childhood. Many hyperactive children fall into this category. They frequently will respond well with medication. With appropriate medication, their activity level is normal, they can sit still when necessary, and secondary emotional problems are prevented from developing.

Of course, individuals with mental retardation or organic brain syndrome should be referred. An individual with an incapacitating neurosis (can't sleep or function socially and biologically) may need referral. Individuals with apparent physical problems (instant blindness or paralysis) should be referred.

Perhaps the question of when to refer could be simplified by listing six classifications that summarize many of the cases needing referral. They are:

1. Refer anyone suicidal. Remember that many people who are extremely depressed are also suicidal.
2. Refer anyone homicidal.
3. Refer anyone with a problem that is beyond the minister's ability and/or whom he feels uncomfortable trying to handle.
4. Refer anyone who is psychotic or manic.
5. Refer anyone who is organic (e.g., delirious, grossly confused, or in drug/alcohol withdrawal) or who has a medical problem that is adversely affecting his or her mental status.
6. Refer anyone when the minister cannot handle the case adequately because of a lack of time in his schedule.

The above list is not comprehensive but does indicate the type of problems that need to be referred. Of course, a basic question in considering referral is whether the problem is spiritual, mental, or physical. We personally believe this line is hard to draw at times. For example, under stress many Christians choose not (or just do not know *how*) to turn to the Lord for help. Thus, the stress increases and mental symptoms develop. Is this a spiritual or mental problem? Certainly, both are involved.

Referrals may be from a minister to a psychiatrist, a psychologist, or an individual in another field. A referral may be from any one of the above to any other of the above. This was discussed in chapter 1. However, we feel that it would be helpful to mention one other point. We have found that when treating a counselee referred by a minister, a brief phone call periodically to keep each other informed can be of much help to the counselee.

Christian Psychiatry—Does It Exist?

Christian psychiatry—does it exist? We believe it does, and we have attempted in this book to present an integration of sound theology with valid psychiatric knowledge into concepts known simply as Christian Psychiatry. We have enjoyed collaborating in the writing of this book and hope the reader has benefited from it.

SOURCE NOTES

Chapter 1

1. Robert Shannon, Lecture on Psychodynamics, University of Arkansas Medical Center, 1972.
2. Solomon and Patch, *Handbook*.
3. Calvin S. Hall and Gardner Lindzey, *Theories of Personality* (New York: John Wiley and Sons, Inc., 1957).
4. Ibid.
5. Ibid.
6. Ibid.
7. Gary Collins, "The Pulpit and the Couch," *Christianity Today* 19 (August 1975): 5–9.
8. Hall and Lindzey, *Theories*.
9. A. M. Nicoli, "A New Dimension of the Youth Culture," *American Journal of Psychiatry* 131 (1974): 396–401.
10. W. P. Wilson, "Mental Health Benefits of Religious Salvation," *Diseases of the Nervous System* 33 (1972): 382–386.
11. C. Christensen, "Religious Conversion," *Archives of General Psychiatry* 9 (1963): 207–216.
12. E. M. Pattison, "Social and Psychological Aspects of Religion in Psychotherapy," *Journal of Nervous and Mental Diseases* 141 (1965): 586–597.
13. S. Janus and B. Bess, "Drug Abuse, Sexual Attitudes, Political Radicalization, and Religious Practices of College Seniors and Public School Teachers," *American Journal of Psychotherapy* 130 (1973): 187–191.
14. L. Allison, "Adaptive Regression and Intense Religious Experiences," *Journal of Nervous and Mental Diseases* 145 (1967): 452–463.

15. S. Freud, "The Future of an Illusion" (1927), in *Complete Psychological Works*, standard ed. 21, trans. J. Strachey (London: Hobarth Press, 1961), 5–56.

16. S. Freud, "Obsessive Actions and Religious Practice" (1907), Ibid. 9: 117–127.

17. S. Freud, "Totem and Taboo" (1912), Ibid. 13: 1–161.

18. W. P. Wilson, "The Religious Life of Patients with Affective Disorders," *Diseases of the Nervous System* 30 (1969): 438–486.

19. B. G. Meyerson and L. Staller, "A Psychoanalytical Interpretation of the Crucifixion," *Psychoanalysis* 49 (4) 1962: 117, 118.

20. P. Bergman, "A Religious Conversion in the Course of Psychotherapy," *American Journal of Psychotherapy* 7 (1953): 41–58.

21. A. Bronner, "Psychotherapy with Religious Patients," *American Journal of Psychotherapy* 18 (1964): 475–487.

22. C. G. Jung, *Mysterium Coniunctionis* 14, trans. R. Hull (New York: Bollingen Foundation, Inc., 1963).

23. E. Fromm, *Escape from Freedom* (New York and Boston: Rinehart and Co., Inc., 1941).

24. A. Adler, *The Individual Psychology of Alfred Adler*, ed. and annotated by Ansbacher and Ansbacher (New York: Basic Books, Inc., 1956): 460–464.

25. W. James, *The Varieties of Religious Experience* (New York: Collier Books, 1961).

26. S. Freud, "Obsessive Actions and Religious Practice."

27. C. G. Jung, *Mysterium Coniunctionis.*

28. W. James, *Varieties.*

29. A. Adler, *The Individual Psychology.*

30. E. Fromm, *Escape From Freedom.*

31. C. Christensen, "Religious Conversion."

32. L. Allison, "Adaptive Regression."

33. E. M. Pattison, "Social and Psychological Aspects of Religion in Psychotherapy."

34. A. Bronner, "Psychotherapy with Religious Patients."

35. P. Bergman, "A Religious Conversion."

36. B. G. Meyerson and L. Staller, "A Psychoanalytical Interpretation of the Crucifixion."

37. W. P. Wilson, "Mental Health Benefits of Religiou˙ Salvation," *Diseases of the Nervous System* 33 (1972): 382–386.

38. W. P. Wilson, "The Religious Life of Patienrͨ with Affective Disorders."

39. A. M. Nicoli, "A New Dimension."

40. Gary Collins, "The Pulpit and the Couch."
41. Ibid.
42. Ibid.
43. Howard Hendricks, "Counseling," Lecture at Dallas Theological Seminary, Dallas, Texas, 1970.
44. Doug Wilson, "A Fresh Perspective on Biblical Counseling," unpublished, December 1975.
45. W. E. Vine, *Expository Dictionary of New Testament Words* (Old Tappan, New Jersey: Fleming Revell Co., 1966).

Chapter 2

1. Paul Tournier, *Guilt and Grace* (New York: Harper & Row, 1962).
2. W. E. Vine, *Expository Dictionary*.
3. *The American College Dictionary*, 1963, s.v. "debt," "works," "law."
4. Lewis Sperry Chafer, *Grace* (Grand Rapids, Michigan: Zondervan Publishing House, 1922).
5. Lewis S. Chafer, *Salvation* (Grand Rapids, Michigan: Zondervan Publishing House, 1917).
6. Lewis S. Chafer, *True Evangelism* (Grand Rapids, Michigan. Zondervan Publishing House, 1967).
7. Harry Ironside, *Full Assurance* (Chicago: Moody Press, 1937)
8. Watchman Nee, *Sit, Walk, Stand* (Fort Washington, Pennsylvania: Christian Literature Crusade, 1957).
9. C. I. Scofield, "Scofield Notes on Galatians," *Scofield Reference Bible* (New York: Oxford University Press, 1945).
10. Charles Haddon Spurgeon, *Spurgeon Sermon Notes* (Grand Rapids, Michigan: Zondervan Publishing House, 1957).
11. Paul Tournier, *Guilt and Grace.*

Chapter 3

1. Lewis S. Chafer, *Systematic Theology* II (Dallas, Texas: Dallas Seminary Press, 1947).
2. Bill Gothard, Basic Youth Conflicts Seminar (Kansas City, November 1972).
3. Charles Hodge, *Systematic Theology* II (New York: Charles Scribner's Sons, 1871).
4. Witness Lee, "Spirit, Soul, and Body," *The Stream* 4:1 (1966).

5. Don Meredith et al., Christian Family Life Seminar (Dallas, Texas, June 1973).

6. Watchman Nee, *The Spiritual Man* I (New York: Christian Fellowship Publishers, Inc., 1968).

7. Augustus H. Strong, *Systematic Theology* (New York: A. C. Armstrong and Son, 1886).

8. W. E. Vine, *Expository Dictionary.*

• 9. Leonard L. Heston, "The Genetics of Schizophrenia."

Chapter 4

1. Thomas P. Detre and Henry G. Jarecki, *Modern Psychiatric Treatment* (Philadelphia: J. B. Lippincott Company, 1971).

2. Clarence W. Rowe, M.D., *An Outline of Psychiatry*, 9th Edition (Dubuque, Iowa: W. C. Brown Publishers, 1989).

3. Detre and Jarecki, *Modern Psychiatric Treatment*

4. Rowe, *An Outline of Psychiatry.*

5. *The Psychiatric Times*, Volume 6, No 10, October 1989, p. 38, Robert G. Robinson, M.D

6. *Diagnostic and Statistical Manual of Mental Disorders*, 3d Edition, Revised (Washington, D.C.. American Psychiatric Association, 1987) p. 85.

7. Ibid.

8. Harold I. Kaplan and Alfred M. Freedman, *Comprehensive Textbook of Psychiatry* (Baltimore: Colan, Williams and Wilkins Company, 1967).

9. *Diagnostic and Statistical Manual of Mental Disorders*, p. 51.

10. Ibid., p. 66.

11. Robert Hemfelt, Frank Minirth, and Paul Meier, *Love Is a Choice* (Nashville: Thomas Nelson, Inc., 1989), p. 28.

12. Ibid.

13. Beulah C. Bosselman, *Neurosis and Psychosis*, 3d Edition (Springfield, Illinois: C. C. Thomas, 1969).

14. J. R. Smythies et al., *Biological Psychiatry: A Review of Ancient Advances* (New York: Springer-Verlag, Inc., 1968).

Chapter 5

1. Manual for the Psychiatry Department of the University of the Arkansas Medical Center, Little Rock, Arkansas, 1972.

Chapter 6

1. Marcus A. Krupp and Milton J. Chatton, *Current Diagnosis and Treatment* (California: Lange Medical Publications, 1973).

Chapter 7

1. Harold I. Kaplan and Alfred M. Freedman, *Comprehensive Testbook*
2. Silvano Arieti et al., eds., *American Handbook of Psychiatry*, 2d ed. (New York: Basic Books, Inc., 1974).
3. Merril Eaton and Margaret Peterson, *Psychiatry.*
4. Lawrence C. Kolb, *Modern Clinical Psychiatry* (Philadelphia: W B. Saunders Company, 1973).
5. Solomon and Patch, *Handbook.*
6. Shannon and Backus, "Depression," *The Journal of the Arkansas Medical Society,* July 1973.
7. S. Arieti et al., eds., *American Handbook of Psychiatry.*
8. Shannon and Backus, "Depression."
9. Ibid.
10. Sir Denis Hill and Lee E. Hollister, eds., *Depression* (Wisconsin: Lakeside Laboratories, Inc., 1970).
11. Shannon and Backus, "Depression."
12. Ibid.
13. W. G. Reese, "The Major Cause of Death," *Texas Medicine* 66, September 1970.
14. Solomon and Patch, *Handbook.*
15. Harold I. Kaplan and Benjamin Sadock, *Clinical Psychiatry* from *Synopsis of Psychiatry* (Baltimore: Williams & Wilkins, 1988), 302–305.
16. Bill Gothard, Basic Youth Conflicts
17. Chuck Singletary, Lecture on the Anatomy of Discouragement (Memphis, 1970).
18. Watchman Nee, *Song of Songs* (Fort Washington, Pennsylvania: Christian Literature Crusade, 1965).
19. Chuck Singletary, Lecture on the Anatomy of Discouragement.
20. Shannon and Backus, "The Psychodynamics of Depression," *Journal of the Arkansas Medical Society,* December 1973.
21. Ibid.
22. W. K. Zung, "The Pharmacology of Disordered Sleep," *Journal of the American Medical Association* 211: March 2, 1970.

23. William Glasser, *Reality Therapy* (New York: Harper & Row, 1965).

24. Harry Ironside, *Full Assurance* (Chicago: Moody Press).

25. William Glasser, *Reality Therapy.*

Chapter 8

1. E. M. Berman and H. I. Lief, "Marital Therapy from a Psychiatric Perspective: An Overview," *American Journal of Psychiatry* 132, No. 6 (June 1975), 583–592.

Chapter 10

1. Eugen Blueler, *Dementia Praecox or the Group of Schizophrenias* (New York: International Universities, 1966).

2. Jerry Blaylock, "Psychopharmacology," unpublished (University of Arkansas Medical Center, 1972).

3. *Drug Treatment in Psychiatry*, Staff of Central NP Research Laboratory, Veterans Administration Hospital, Perry Point, Maryland (Washington, D.C.: Veterans Administration).

4. Marcus A. Krupp and Milton J. Chatton, *Current Diagnosis and Treatment.*

5. Robert Shannon, Lecture on Psychodynamics, unpublished (University of Arkansas Medical Center, 1972).

6. Solomon and Patch, *Handbook.*

7. J. R. Smythies, *Biological Psychiatry.*

8. A. Schatzberg, M.D., and J. Cole, M.D., *Manual of Clinical Psychopharmacology*, American Psychiatric Press (Washington, D.C., 1986).

Chapter 11

1. Thomas A. Harris, *I'm OK—You're OK: A Practical Guide to* TA (New York: Harper & Row, 1969).

2. Kenneth F. Weaver, "The Incredible Universe," *National Geographic* 145 (1974): 589–625.

3. "Seven Minutes With God" (Colorado Springs: Navigators).

4. Glasser, *Reality Therapy.*

Chapter 12

1. Cyrus T. Scofield, "Scofield Notes on Job," *Scofield Reference Bible* (New York: Oxford University Press, 1909).

Index

Child: as counselee, 124; in TA, 48–49.
See also Childhood
Childhood: autistic disorder, 95–96; pervasive developmental disorder of, 95
Chlorpromazine, 175
Christ: as directive, 164; counseling approach of, 166; as counselor, 206, 211–212; in us, 41–42; purpose for, 200; simplicity of, 39–40. *See also* God
Christensen, C., 23
Christian counseling: balance needed in, 30–31; defined, 25; theology of healthy, 33–46; therapeutic steps in, 201–207; uniqueness of, 25–29. *See also* Christian counselor
Christian counselor: categories of, 23–25; character of, 190–201; characteristics of, 191–198; qualities of, 198–201
Christian professional, 24
Christian psychiatry: and psychoanalysis, 47–59; and transactional analysis, 47–59
Chronic motor/vocal tic disorder, 101
Clinical pastoral education (CPE) movement, 23–24
Cluttering, 102
Co-dependency, 115
Co-dependent, traits of, 115–116
Cognitive therapy, 17, 20
Collins, Gary, 23–25
Communication, as parameter, 125–126
Compensation, as defense mechanism, 87
Compulsions, 105–106
Confession, prayer as, 196
Confidence, and good counseling, 201
Confronting, and good counseling, 199
Conscience: in depressive counselees, 134–135; lack of, in sociopathic man, 156; and "parent," 51; and Spirit, 49–50; as standard of authority, 21–22; and superego, 51. *See also* Conscience, Christian
Conscience, Christian: factors in, 56–57; vs. non-Christian, 50
Conversion, changes due to, 57–58
Conversion type: hysterical neurosis, 99; somatoform disorder of, 99
Counseling: directive vs. non-directive, 163–166; indirect-directive, 163–173; principles in, 163; as profession, 16. *See also* Christian counseling

Counseling process, 166, 169
Counselling for Substance Abuse and Addiction (Van Cleave, Boyd, and Revell), 117
Cross, psychoanalytic meaning of, 23
Cyclothymic personality, 83

David, King, 86, 138, 142, 148, 165–166, 192, 203
Debt, grace vs., 35
Decision-making process, 173
Defense mechanisms, 85–88
Delusional thinking, 136
Delusions, and need for professional help, 213
Dementia: symptoms of, 97–98. *See also* Organic brain syndrome
Demon possession, and obsessive-compulsive problem, 109–110
Demonic influences, 171
Denial, 21
Dependent personality disorder, 77–78
Depersonalization disorder, 104
Depression: biblical mention of, 65; causes of, 137–146; dealing with, 146–149; medications for, 176–179, 185–186; occurrence of, 136; symptoms of, 133–136
Detre, Thomas, 63
Diagnostic and Statistical Manual (DSM III-R), 73
Dicks, Russell, 24
Directive counseling, 163–166
Disorganized schizophrenia, 94
Displacement, 87
Disulfiram (Antabuse), 181
Double-bind message: damage of, 33–34; grace and, 33–46
Drugs: and referrals, 182; used in psychiatry, 174–189. *See also* Medications
Dynamic formulation, 127

Early parental teaching, and conscience, 21–22, 56, 57
Ego, 17
Ego boundaries, loss of, 91
Ego states, TA, 19
Elective mutism, 102
Electroconvulsive therapy (ECT), 178
Elihu, 164, 199, 208–210
Elijah, 138
Eliphaz, 209
Ellis, Albert, 20